Yoga Philosophy

Essential Yoga Poses to Transform Your Mind,
Body & Spirit

(A Beginner's Guide to Lose Weight, Obtain
Mental Clarity & Find True Focus)

Jessamyn Hollister

Published by Rob Miles

Jessamyn Hollister

Yoga Philosophy: Essential Yoga Poses to Transform Your Mind, Body & Spirit (A Beginner's Guide to Lose Weight, Obtain Mental Clarity & Find True Focus)

ISBN 978-1-989990-59-9

Legal & Disclaimer

The information contained in this book is not designed to replace or take the place of any form of medicine or professional medical advice. The information in this book has been provided for educational and entertainment purposes only.

The information contained in this book has been compiled from sources deemed reliable, and it is accurate to the best of the Author's knowledge; however, the Author cannot guarantee its accuracy and validity and cannot be held liable for any errors or omissions. Changes are periodically made to this book. You must consult your doctor or get professional medical advice before using any of the suggested remedies, techniques, or information in this book.

Table of Contents

It is a science, the science of well-being, youthfulness, integrating body, mind, and soul. The practice of Yoga aligns your body, mind and soul, keeps you mentally and physically fit, and helps you explore yourself in a better manner.

However, what exactly is yoga? How can you practice it, and how does it benefit you? These common questions pop into our mind whenever we hear someone rambling on about the amazingness of yoga.

This book seeks to answer these questions,as well as provide you with a step-by-step guide on how best to integrate various beneficial yoga poses into your everyday life and in the process, enhance your quality of life.

Let us begin our journey into yoga and your practice of it by gaining an in-depth insight of yoga as a mind and body practice.

Thanks again for downloading this book, I hope you enjoy it!

CHAPTER 1: YIN YOGA: THE CONCEPT DEFINED

What is Yin Yoga? I have asked this question myself when I came across this term. While I am familiar with Hatha, Bikram, and Ashtanga yoga, I had never practiced this style before. Many of you might also have the same question.

To put in simple words, Yin Yoga is exactly the opposite of a classical Hatha or Ashtanga practice. While the goals and intentions are the same, the way of practice is pretty inactive. It complements the dynamic Yoga styles which most of us are practicing at the moment. While the Yang style [the other practices] work on raising our metabolism by generating internal heat, Yin calms the agitated muscles.

As I mentioned above, even though its goals match with the Yang practices, the focus of Yin Yoga is entirely different. It concentrates on the underlying deep tissues, the joints, and ligaments which generally do not receive attention in the active styles.

Hips, lower spine, knees, and pelvis are the areas that receive more attention. But, yes, there are individual flows those cater to the needs of shoulders, neck, and upper back as well.

This style of yoga looks pretty simple, but when you practice you feel the challenge. Holding a posture for 5 to 6 minutes without movements... the practice, indeed, teaches you patience.

So, how different is Yin from other practices? Let's take a closer look!

How is it different from other yoga practices?

If you have been practicing Hatha or any other active style of Yoga for a while now, you will realize that the center of attention is purely muscular. Perfect alignment is what makes these practices come alive. In those methods, you, in fact, force your body to get into a stretch to feel the burn.

On the other hand, Yin Yoga looks more into the underlying and softer parts of the human body. You do not push yourself here. The focus is on disengaging the muscle. The aim is to build flexibility without hurting the body.

There are three major elements when it comes to a Yin practice:

☐Come to your edge while getting into a pose

☐Hold the pose for a long duration (5 minutes is the minimum)

☐Remain in stillness

We love movement while holding Asanas, adjusting ourselves to get the alignment right. It is tough to remain still.

That could be the reason why props are used widely in Yin practices. Props instill a sense of comfort, helping you breathe into the poses and hold them while resorting to a sense of inner peace and calmness. Your muscles experience a sense of relief as you do not have to burn your stamina to hold a particular pose.

There are no Warriors, Backbends Inversions, or Arm Balances. The majority of poses are seated or reclining. Of course, there are times when we do a Downward Facing Dog pose for a couple of minutes, but to release the tension. Dangling with bent knees, a variation of Uttanasana (Standing Forward Fold), is also used as release posture.

We'll look deeper into these as we go through the poses and flows...

For now, let's take a walk down the memory lane of Yin Yoga!

History of Yin Yoga

Yoga, in the ancient days, was pretty similar to the Yin Yoga with the poses being held for prolonged periods. As time changed, there was a shift in the demands of the world which led to the popularization of the active, Yang poses. But, Mother Nature always sweeps her magic wand when She knows that it is time to restore the natural balance.

That happened with Yoga also. Sometime during the late 1980s, two Yogis began to restore this balance. The two Yogis were named Paul Grilley and Sarah Powers.

Paul's first stint with this type of Yoga happened when he visited Paulie Zink's Daoist Yoga. Paulie was a martial art teacher who used to hold stretches for about 30 minutes. While Paulie's classes offered both the styles, it was Yin that caught Paul's attention. He was a yoga teacher already during that time.

He decided to create a class which comprised only the seated postures. He was able to achieve that inner balance he was yearning and searching. But, Yin Yoga was not so straightforward and easy to achieve as it looked. It actually carved an opportunity for Paul's students to explore a realm that they have never ventured before.

Sarah was Paul's student along with being a teacher. As Paul explained the importance of these postures, Sarah felt the urge to learn more about these postures. And, in the process, both of them started on a journey of creating the masterpiece called Yin Yoga.

Sarah christened the practice as Yin Yoga by Sarah, as it involved seated postures. She, by then, had introduced her students to this practice, allowing them to immerse in a new state of tranquility through this meditative practice.

Yin Yoga slowly spread across the world with the students of Sarah and Paul handing them over to their students. It was through one of their pupils, Bernie Clark, that the style gained popularity.

And now...

It is time for you to experience the stillness of Yin Yoga. It is natural that we do not all have the patience to sit in a place without fidgeting. It is as if we are trying to run away from something… much as we do in our daily lives. Instead of facing a challenge with courage, we try to overlook or run away from it.

Distraction is a game our monkey mind plays. It just loves to run and hop around, delving into the past and wandering into the future. It tempts you to leave the present. So, why not challenge the mind? You are its master and not vice versa.

Challenge and woo your mind with a new dose of patience with Yin Yoga. Do not expect miracles to happen with the first attempt. You are bound to experience how still you are when you fold forward or recline. You will experience the difference between your left and right sides. But do not worry!

All you have to do is just to breathe, observe, accept, and surrender! Restore that lost friendship among your body, mind, and soul with Yin Yoga!

In the further chapters, we'll explore a little more about the Yin and Yang concepts, benefits of practicing this style of yoga, what all do you need to practice it, the various asanas, and some flows….

Take one step at a time… Try holding one posture at a time…As you learn how to remain still, you can try practicing the flows…

We lay on the ground, stomach up, thighs somewhat apart, hands at your edges and palms facing up. The whole body remains motionless and you can freely relax every muscle.

Typically, we'd have our eyes closed, but in a technique that is attentive and conscious, we abstract ourselves from worry or any negative thought, and we focus on the teacher's style. To accomplish relaxation of body and intellect, in addition to enjoyable looks or music, the gradual pace through breathing practices, required by the teacher, leads us from toenails, in a progressive relaxation of the complete body towards the tips of the hair.

By the end of a yoga class and now ultimate exercise, you calm your ideas, the breath flows slowly but deeply, heart beats' volume gets lower, and there's a launch of hormones.

11

The feel is being more powerful yet relaxed. We feel rejuvenated. The most fanatical professionals of meditation or yoga will state that this method is a 'pure large.'

Not being a physician of yoga you're able to - and should - try this method of peace. The advantages could be more powerful if you do it at the end of a period of yoga but works great if you want to relax even before doing any yoga position.

Since the accomplishment of this exercise requires the capability to focus, the snowball effect begins within the intellect. You simply need to remember it, when you can realize the specified, within the next situations. The body learns to activate this anti-anxiety process simply by considering it, and you can stimulate it.

Yoga is a good exercise that releases tension and creates power within your body. It also helps your body conduct at its highest potential. Yoga feels that human beings are registered with character.

Therefore being normally healthy provides you closer to nature.

You'll find proven benefits of yoga, it increases freedom, helps muscles and your energy. Additionally, it may help your body build a stronger immune system by getting the appropriate exercise and delivering toxins in your body. Yoga advances characteristics of your lungs and the quality of your breathing with basic breathing techniques. Yoga will help you get healthy literally and mentally, by relieving tension, depression and bodily injuries all at the same time.

If weight reduction is your purpose you then can simply benefit from doing yoga. Yoga improves your body physically equally as it will psychologically, it will help burn fat and tighten your muscles. Consequently creating yoga a powerful exercise that anyone may do. Yoga is usually discussed being a psychological exercise, but there are lots of proven physical benefits of doing yoga regularly. Yoga is protected for elders. Also, it will help improve and cure bones and structures.

Yoga helps to launch negative electricity which all results in a healthier lifestyle, and cleanses your body of daily toxins. Yoga has become extremely popular all over the planet, rendering it available to anyone who would like to see and to study the advantages and has awesome benefits.

You can study Yoga without leaving your home; an extensive variety of home videos and online education is available. You get yourself an individual trainer if you want or can also join yoga courses, it-all-depends on specifications and your lifestyle. Produce some time for yourself and give yoga a try, and experience the wonderful benefits yourself.

Simple yoga exercises, breathing methods, and leisure techniques are some of the very popular ways of relaxing.

Similar to people, you may spend every day busy at work, you invest energy and time to accomplish your absolute best and provide your best to work colleagues, family and friends.

Most of the time you probably enjoy life, you have a wide cultural network, whether it is an online area, like Facebook or friends that you meet outside of work. You appreciate health and are informed of eating properly and of the pros and cons.

In most cases you feel satisfied and content with life. When anything goes wrong if this seems like you, how can you deal? For example, imagine your spouse instantly falls ill, and you also need to accept the elephants' share of domestic duties and care for your young children; maybe you happen to be promoted at your job, therefore, you need to spend more time on the street traveling between consumers and less time aware of your household.

Change, whether negative or positive is tense. No matter when you are faced with unexpected changes to your everyday regime, how balanced or good you are about living, the body acts and strains resulting in anxiety build ups.

You are not sure what direction to go, and while life extends you, a good thing you can certainly do is relax. Just a couple moments of relaxation exercises can give you the chance to re-evaluate and rethink your choices available to you.

Listed here are my four of my favorite yoga practices that you can use to guide you and release strain if you have challenging choices to make.

Top Four Yoga Techniques to Allow You To Release Tension

1. Yoga exercises help you to stretch and release anxiety and tension energy located in your body. The absence of exercise is just a contributory element in several stress-related health issues, particularly

while you grow older. Easy exercises, accomplished a few times through your day helps you to find comfort and also to bolster your system and make it more flexible.

2. Yoga breathing exercises will give you a basic and efficient approach to relieving tension, particularly from what I call short-term stress situations, for example, needing to give a report to your boss today but your child is unwell which means you feel too exhausted to complete the investigation and produce the record.

When you feel stressed and exhausted, spend 2 - 5 minutes taking note of the motion of breath, first of your neck, back throughout your nose and all the way down to your belly, just be still and discover your breathing. At the conclusion of the exercise, you'll be surprised at how refocused you are feeling and how much clearer and energized you are.

3. Yoga techniques. Through yoga, inner peace is experienced. While you reflect

you experience a greater perception of body consciousness, you recognize where you carry stress and stiffness, where the fluctuations are in the human body. So you do not yield so quickly to stressful situations, an everyday yoga practice builds up your inner reservoirs.

4. Yoga diet. A healthy diet, one who is abundant with wholesome and live food offers the human body with the enzymes and vitamins needed to build up and keep powerful defense mechanisms. When you are dealing with a stressful time try and eat a broad array of greens and snack on fruits.

CHAPTER 3: WHY PRACTICE YOGA?

If you would like to be healthier then you want to practice yoga. Yoga strengthens your body and mind. It can also help relieve the symptoms of some physical and mental diseases.

Yoga can also sculpt your body, enhance your sexual health and it can also help you sleep better.

Here are some of the reasons why you should practice yoga:

1. Yoga relieves stress.

These days everyone seems to be working too hard and so stress is inevitable. Yoga helps relieve stress and it helps ease anxiety because of its calming effect.

2. Yoga is a holistic exercise.

Many people try different forms of exercise including dancing, biking and jogging. These exercises help release endorphins from your body. Infact, yoga is a total body workout that uses a holistic approach. It enables you to stretch out your muscles. It builds your abdomen and also tones your buttocks, legs and arms- yoga makes you more flexible and stronger.

Yoga is also flexible- meaning you can exercise at your own pace. It is an amazing mix of strength and cardio training.

3. Yoga improves your posture.

You exude confidence when you have a good posture. Yoga improves your posture because it allows you to stretch and tone your muscles, thus making them stronger.

4. Yoga has different health benefits.

Yoga has many health benefits. It can ease migraines and other forms of headache. For instance, Sirsasana or Headstand is a yoga pose that increases the oxygen flow in your brain to help relieve headaches.

Yoga also boosts your immune system thanks to its many biochemical benefits. The regular practice of yoga decreases your cholesterol and glucose level. It also increases your hemoglobin count .It also decreases the production of stress hormone called cortisol and it increases the production of happy hormones called endorphins.

5. Yoga improves your flexibility.

When you practice yoga regularly you become more flexible. As a result, it is easier for you to do chores. This will increase your productivity.

6. Yoga enhances your sexual health.

Practicing yoga regularly will improve your sexual health and it will also improve your fertility. Women who are having a hard time conceiving should try yoga.

7. Yoga helps you sleep better.

Yoga helps ease insomnia and other sleep disorders. Many sleep doctors recommend yoga to their patients to help them relax and enable them to get some quality sleep.

8. Yoga can improve your mental health.

Yoga is also popular because of its ability to heal deep-seated emotional wounds. It also improves your overall psychological health. The regular practice of yoga can actually helps relieve depression, eases anxiety and help manage stress. It also increases your social skills, self-esteem and self-confidence. As well,it can also helps develop social acceptance and helps you manage your mood.

9. Yoga helps you lose weight

This is probably the reason why yoga is practiced by many fitness enthusiasts. Yoga can help you lose weight in four different ways:

☐ It helps cleanse your colon or large intestine.

Yoga has a detoxifying effect. It cleanses your colon and it increases your metabolism. It also helps eliminate digestive problems.

☐It activates your thyroid gland.

Your thyroid gland regulates your metabolism. When your thyroid gland is not functioning well your metabolism is slower and it will be harder for you to burn fats. Many yoga poses help activate your thyroid gland and increase your metabolism.

☐It improves your liver function.

Yoga cleanses and strengthens your liver. If you have a healthy liver then it is easier to lose weight.

☐It creates nerve tension.

Yoga helps you lose weight by activating heat in your nervous system. This helps you purify and burn fats.

☐It burns fats and builds your muscle.

Certain yoga poses can help you burn fats. Many yoga poses also build and tone your muscles.

Yoga transforms your body and mind. It is a holistic discipline. It does not only help you manage your weight and tone your body- it also helps you become healthier, stronger and live a happier and a more fulfilling life.

Not all forms of yoga are the same. You need to choose the type of yoga that works best for you; choose the one that is in line with your fitness and health goals.

1. Hatha yoga is the yoga practice that helps you get acquainted with the very basic yoga poses. You will learn proper breathing, yoga poses and basic meditation in a Hatha yoga class.

2. Ashtanga yoga is fast paced and very athletic. It is generally made up of six complicated and strenuous sequence of yoga postures. It is one of the oldest types of yoga. It is also the type of yoga usually taught in Western countries. In fact, most gyms in Western countries teach Ashtanga yoga. This type of yoga is also perfect for weight loss because it burns a lot of calories. Ashtanga yoga also tones your body and builds your muscle.

3. Most fitness enthusiasts choose this type of yoga practice because it optimizes the weight loss benefits of yoga. Bikram yoga is done in a heated room to help burn fat more easily and it helps detoxify the body.

4. This is one of the advanced forms of yoga. The goal of this yoga practice is to awaken the kundalini energy located at the end of your spine. Once you have activated your kundalini energy all your chakras will open. Activating your kundalini energy will detoxify your mind and it will enhance your cognitive function. People who practice Kundalini yoga feel enlightened and happy.

5. This is a fusion of Hatha and Ashtanga yoga. It groups and links certain asanas to make a good sequence. Restorative yoga is generally used by people who are recovering from accidents. It is also used by older individuals who are suffering from different health problems.

6. ⬚⬚⬚⬚⬚⬚⬚⬚⬚⬚⬚⬚⬚

This form of yoga is often called the Westernized yoga. It concentrates on breathing and balance. This type of yoga practice could be challenging for beginners.

7. Vinyasa yoga was derived from Ashtanga. It is a rhythmic and steady flow of poses. Classes focus on the natural and genuine movement of the body. It is also meditative. From Hatha yoga, you can transition to Vinyasa if you are looking for a little bit of a challenge.

Yoga is a great tool for weight loss. But, more than that, yoga transforms your body, mind, and spirit. It transforms the way you look at your body. It change the way you think and the way you look at life. Yoga helps you become fitter, happier and more grounded.

Chapter 5: Introduction To The Mudras And Basic Poses

In the ancient Yoga Sutras of Patanjali, physical postures constitute one of eight limbs of yoga. The other limbs deal with breathing, conduct and the power of the mind that will help in bringing out your divine inner qualities, which you can apply in your everyday life.

This book focuses on the two practices of the physical aspect of yoga – mudras and asanas. How do these two concepts help in giving you a healthy physical and emotional state? How do you gain benefits from the practice?

Yoga practice is all about who you are from within. It serves as a medium for you to bring out and understand your core. It helps you to naturally evolve to the higher stages of understanding and living life.

Every human being has a physical and non-physical existence, all of which are composed of different layers. Yoga is geared towards the opening or activating of the principles that will hone each layer that is found within you. The physical practices of yoga are dealt with by learning more about asanas, mudras and bandhas.

Bandhas are physical, but most of the time, are static poses that are aimed at the areas of the body that hinder the flow of neurobiological energies from deep within. With the help of the practice, you will be able to direct the energy to flow in the right direction and to where it is needed.

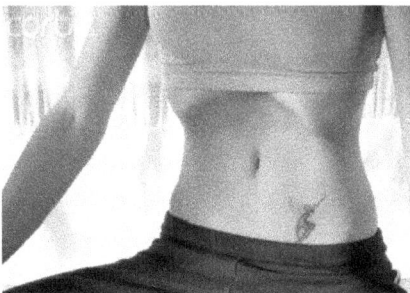

Asanas refer to the physical poses, postures and seats that you will learn how to cultivate in order to improve the spiritual growth of your nervous system, especially the central spinal nerve.

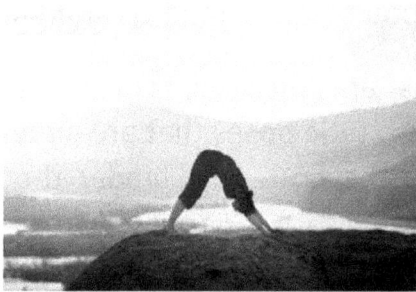

Mudras are composed of physical and, at times, dynamic poses that are geared towards the areas of your system that seal or channel the flow of the neurobiological energies from your core.

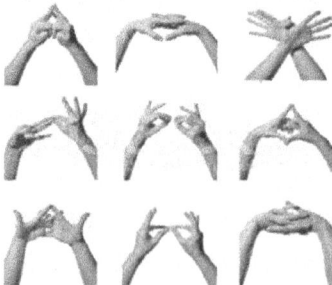

Among the three concepts, asanas are more known worldwide and are actually being integrated in various exercises and physical fitness activities. This is a good thing because it keeps the interests of many people in yoga. This is only the beginning. Once you have mastered the right poses, it is only natural to find out more about the concept and how you can benefit from it. This leads to finding out more about the other yoga methods, breathing techniques and practices.

Mudras and bandhas are separate practices with similarities and overlaps. Both concepts are inward when it comes to appearance and performance. They both train the natural physical processes deep within you until you have reached the point where you have awakened the Kundalini. This is the point where you will experience spiritual ecstasy.

These concepts - asanas, mudras and bandhas, are the three major ways in yoga in which your physical state and spirit are joined.

Mudras

A mudra is a gesture that is typically done using the hands. As you perform a yoga pose, the mudra directs it to what you ought to focus into. Mudras come in many kinds and they have been used since the ancient times. They are also referred to as seals because the movements involve the connection of the two parts of your hand. The goal is to create prana or pathways for energy by unblocking the chakras.

It is said that mudras have healing effects due to the reflexology points and acupressure that are found in the hands. There are also certain mudras that do not only heal, but are also symbolic in nature. All the aspects of yoga, including mudras, need practice in order to begin benefitting from the techniques.

You cannot treat mudras as a quick fix and expect your problems to go away once you have perfected the pose and sequences. You have to be consistent in practicing the poses and serious in imbibing what this is all about.

In yoga, the fingers and toes are believed to be charged with divine power. Each gesture is called a mudra or seal. It is hand pantomime that is done based on the rituals and carries a visual message that is similar to a hieroglyph.

There are numerous types of mudras that range from simple to complex, types that are performed using one hand and the others that need both hands. After you have mastered the art and principles of hand mudras, you can choose to learn more about the mudras that are made using the eyes or tongue.

When you have completed a mudra, it symbolically means that you have surrendered yourself and you are devoted to what you are doing. When done during pranayama or meditation, the mudra seals the prana, directs it in your entire body and prevents it from leaking out through your fingers. You will notice the big difference after you have completed a mudra. With the fixed hand pose, you will notice that your brain begins to calm and your restless fingers become quiet.

Mudras can be done in any kinds of yoga and you can do the poses anywhere you are. They are best performed when doing relaxation and meditation poses. This is the reason why mudras are integral in Kundalini yoga. It assists in awakening your kundalini. There are practitioners who have experienced the healing powers of mudras.

The Basics about Mudras

Here are the common mudras that are typically used in Hatha yoga. You will be surprised that you may have been doing some of them, but did not know what they are. Some of these mudras will be further explained in the succeeding chapters.

1. Anjali Mudra. This is the most common and is sometimes referred to as the prayer or Namaste position. To perform the pose, firmly press your left palm with your right palm as if you are praying. This simple pose when done right and constantly will bring in calmness in your being. It is perceived to bring the right and left sides of your brain in harmony.

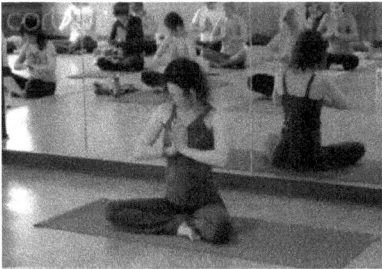

2. Gyan Mudra. Relax your fingers, and then bring your thumb and forefinger closer and press them firmly, leaving the rest of the fingers lying straight. If you are doing this mudra in a cross-legged pose, allow the backs of your hands to comfortably lie on your thighs. This is also

called Jnana mudra or knowledge mudra and it symbolizes connection and oneness.

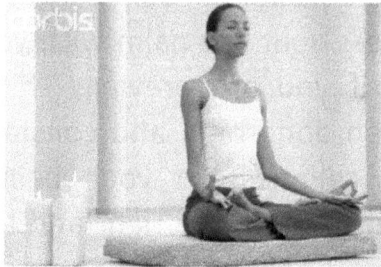

3. Vishnu Mudra. The pose is typically done when performing Nadi Sodhana or alternate nostril breathing. Put your index and middle fingers towards the direction of your palm. While the two fingers are bent, keep the rest of the fingers – the thumb, ring and pinky fingers, extended.

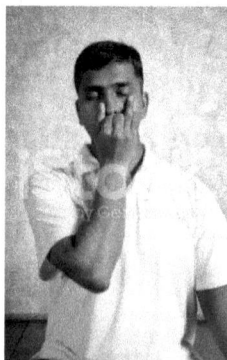

4. Garuda Mudra. This comes from the same origin as the eagle pose or Garudasana, which is said to have a balancing and invigorating effect. The pose is similar to a bird. Cross your wrists with your palms to the direction of your chest. As you do this, hook the thumbs of your two hands together.

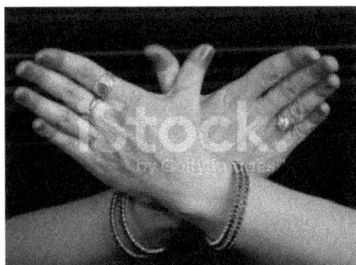

5. Dhyana Mudra. This is considered as a classic Buddhist meditation pose. Relax and sit down, while you lay your left hand on your lap with the palm facing up. Put your right hand on top of the left and as you do this, let your thumbs get in contact above your palms.

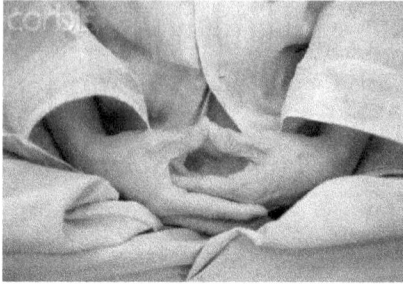

6. Lotus Mudra. Perform the pose that is similar to Anjali mudra, with both of your palms touching. Do not allow your thumbs, pinkies and the bases of your palms to disconnect as you begin to separate the middle parts of your palms and spread the rest of the fingers. Once done, you will notice that the pose is similar to the shape of a lotus flower. Like a flower, this mudra symbolizes openness and blossoming.

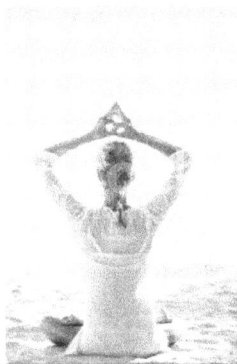

7. Kundalini Mudra. The pose is assimilated with one's sexuality and unity. Form a fist with your left hand, while keeping the index finger extended. Grip that index finger with your right hand as you also make a fist with this hand. Keep the thumb of your right hand lying on top of the index finger of your left hand.

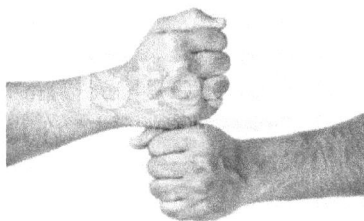

Mastering the Yoga Poses and Mudras for Beginners

In order to consistently practice the mudras, you must also know the right poses that you can perform. Each pose can differ depending on your capabilities, strengths and weaknesses. Here's a look at the common poses that you can start familiarizing yourself with and how to perform the right mudra for each pose.

1. Revolved Lunge

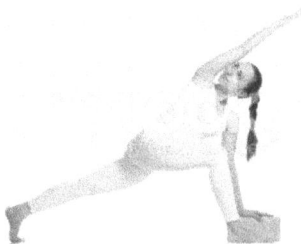

This is a detoxifying pose that requires flexibility, balance and strength. It is detoxifying because you will perform a twist, which in effect, will wring out your internal organs and give your chest enough room to breathe by the end of the pose.

You will begin this by doing a regular lunge. Put your hands down. Twist to the right by stepping your left foot backward. You will end up in a high lunge pose with your knee directly facing your ankle and all your toes are facing forward. Make your weight stable in order to attain balance by reaching through the back heel. At this point, you will bring your hands to Anjali mudra in front of your chest and perform a twist to the right.

Place your elbow and press it outside of the knee. Put your hands together and place them in the middle part of your chest. You may find it hard in the beginning to put your elbow down to your knee. This is only normal and you will eventually get used to it. While you still can't perform the pose properly, you can retain one hand in prayer position while the other arm is extended.

There are also instances when people find it hard to keep their balance. In this case, keep the back of your knee down with your toes tucked underneath. As a beginner, it is more important to keep your lower back safe than to perform the movements perfectly.

You can opt to perform the twist in a low lunge, which means that you will only be twisting your rib cage. Make sure that the belly button is up as you twist. Keep your chin a little bit tucked as you reach the crown of your head. Come out of the pose by coming back to the lunge position with your hands down. Step forward and roll up as gently as you can.

2. Pandangustasana

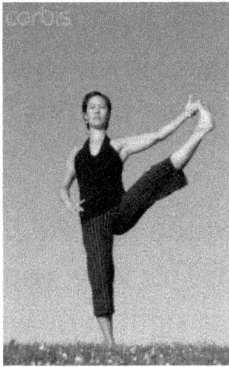

This is also called toe stand and is typically performed in Bikram yoga. This helps in opening the hips and in making the core of the feet stronger. You will begin by standing in a half lotus tree pose. To make it easier for you to do the pose, perform hip stretches before you begin.

This has to be done carefully by those who are having problems with their knees. If the pain continues no matter how careful you are, stop doing the pose and simply look for the poses that are suited for your condition.

Begin by standing on your right leg. Move the top of your left foot towards your right hip. You are now standing in a half lotus tree pose. Maintain your balance by taking several breaths. Slowly bend your right knee while keeping the left foot on top of the left thigh.

As you perform the movement, start lifting your right heel. This way, you will be up on the ball of your right foot when you have reached the squatting position. As you go on a squat, do your best so that the right heel will be in the center of your body. It is a common mistake to aim the right heel under the right buttock.

Once you are in a squat position, extend your fingertips to the floor ahead of you in order to attain more balance. Make your belly firm as you try to lift one hand or both, if you can, off the floor. As you do this, keep your balance on the ball of your right foot.

Once you have achieved the perfect balance, move your hands and perform Anjali mudra. Hold the pose as you inhale and exhale deeply for five counts. You will get out of the pose by rising back to the half lotus tree pose. You will do the same to the other side, but shake both legs first before you continue.

What will you do if you really can't perform the half lotus pose? If your hips find it hard to follow the sequence, focus on attaining your balance in a squat with your heels lifted and your knees together. You will eventually get this right and find it easy. Once you have gotten to this point, you can challenge yourself by coming in and out of the pose without allowing your hands to touch the floor.

3. Skandasana

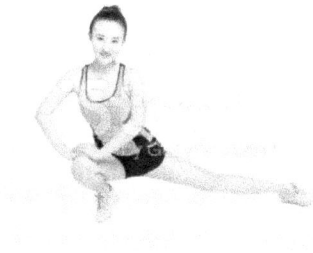

This is also called the deep side lunge. This can be done in a variety of ways. For one, you can perform the pose by having one foot hooked at the back of your head as you are performing a seated forward bend. This can also be done while standing, with the foot still hooked behind the head. This strengthens and exercises your hips and hamstrings, while giving you an improved balance and core strength.

You will begin by doing a wide-legged forward bend or Prasarita Padottanasana. Gently bend your knee until you are doing a half squat. Make sure that your right leg remains straight as you extend your foot and let your toes leave the floor. Rest your weight on your right heel. You can opt to keep your hands on the floor, especially if you are still finding it hard to attain balance.

Once you are already used to it, you can bend your elbows as you bring your hands together to perform an Anjali mudra pose, with your left elbow kept at the inner part of the left knee. When you are ready to come off from the pose, you will simply drop your hands to the floor to get support. You will then shift and perform the actions to the other side.

Beginners are not expected to get into a full squat. It takes practice and getting used to. While you are still trying to perfect the pose, you can stay up on the ball of the left foot.

After familiarizing yourself with the basic and easier poses, you can go ahead and explore the other yoga practices. You will later learn that there are poses that can be modified and certain poses that can be combined, depending on what you want to obtain.

Now that you have performed Cow Pose in which you push your belly and spine downwards, gently move into Cat Pose, which requires pulling your back and abdomen upwards. Cow Pose and Cat Pose are the perfect pairing.

If you have pets at home or even if you have observed them elsewhere, you may be able to visualize how Cat Pose would look like. The name of the pose is equally suggestive. The pose is called Marjariasana in Sanskrit. Marjari means "cat".

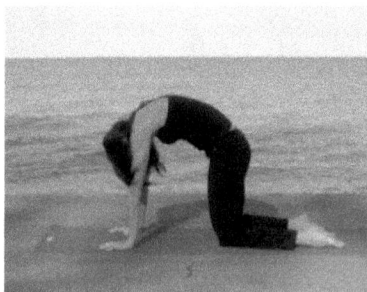

From Cow Pose To Cat Pose

Now you will be coming out of the Cow Pose to Cat Pose. From Cow Pose breathe out as you lift your back to form an arch. Here you go for step-by-step method. When you become more familiar with these techniques, you may performed a Cow - Cat sequence.

How To Do Cat Pose

Come down on fours with your hands and knees on the ground. Let the hands be perpendicular to your shoulders and knees to your hips. Ensure hip-width distance between your knees. Now, you will resemble a tabletop.

Let your head be in neutral position with the gaze fixed on the floor.

Exhale as you lift your back so that the spine is arched as high as possible. Lower the chin towards your chest but not forcibly. Only lower till you are comfortable.

Let the butt be relaxed.

Remain in the pose for few seconds.

Exhale and return to tabletop position.

Repeat the steps 10-20 times or for 1 minute, as slowly as desired.

Don't forget to breathe and try to exhale when releasing.

As mentioned, Cow Pose is often performed with Cat Pose. Doing the poses in a flowing style will relax your back.

Benefits of Cat Pose

Cat Pose has a long list of benefits. The benefits include:

Tones the spine and back muscles

Stretches the back

Corrects wrong posture

Purifies blood and promotes blood circulation

Relieves back pain in pregnant women

Supports pregnancy term and gets pregnant women ready for labor

Tones abdominal organs

Improves digestion

Strengthens wrists

Relieves physical and mental stress

Note

Those with chronic back and neck issues should avoid practicing the pose. If the neck problem is temporary and minor, you may perform the pose with the head in neutral position throughout.

Using Props

A blanket can be placed under the knees if you find it difficult to place your knees on the floor.

CHAPTER 7: SUN SALUTATION

There are many reasons why the Sun Salutation exercises become a staple part of yoga practice. Among these reasons are the following:

☐ It helps the body to celebrate the coming of another day

☐ It helps to strengthen the body

☐ It helps blood to flow and also helps the mind to feel serene

☐ It helps to balance the chakras

☐ It energizes

☐ It teaches students to appreciate humility

☐ It brings much peace to the inner body and reduces depression

There is much more to it, as you will learn as you get more advanced in yoga though, for now, these are very good reasons to perform the exercises. The movements that you perform when you do the Sun Salutation are basic ones. Don't strain your body. The idea is not to hurt yourself. You are a beginner at this stage and it's not about performance. It's about helping your body and mind to come together and to celebrate life.

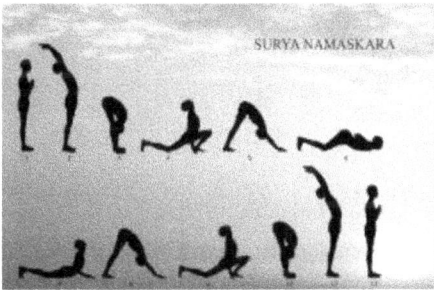

In this image by Surya Namaskara, you can see the movements of the body clearly. These go through a set sequence as you can see in the image and although some of them may seem a little cumbersome at first, you will feel them help balance your body as you perform the exercises.

What is a chakra?

As a beginner, you have probably heard the word "chakra" but you may not realize its significance. The 7 chakras are distributed within the body and account for energy flow. If they are blocked, you can become ill or can suffer injury. The idea of the Sun Salutation is to free up these chakras so that your body feels in tune with movement and is able to become more flexible as a result.

Each of the chakras is located in different parts of the body and for now, all you need to know is that the exercises that you are doing have been designed to help you to feel energetic and well. If your chakras are not in balance, you may be suffering from depression or there may be some sign that all is not right within your body. Thus, balancing the chakras is the ultimate goal of the Sun Salutation exercises.

Why it will help you to learn the Sun Salutation in a class

The support that you gain from doing these exercises in a group is amazing. As a new yoga practitioner, you need to learn the movements and perform them effectively. Thus, if you have a yoga teacher, they will be able to help you and advise you in areas where you experience difficulties. They will also know how to teach you the exercises gradually so that you do not put strain on your body. This, in turn, will improve your flexibility and you will notice that you begin to do the Sun Salutation more naturally once you have been through classes.

Remember, this isn't a sport. There is no competition. Even though you may think that yoga requires you to push yourself to the limits like other sports, that's not the main purpose of yoga. The main purpose is to tune you into your body. That's much more important than simply performing exercises with no awareness of self and balance.

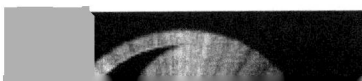

CHAPTER 8: ASHTANGA YOGA

When it comes to Ashtanga yoga, many of its poses are designed to help your detoxify both the mind and body. You may not be aware of it but many of our habits tend to cause an accumulation of toxins in our system. If left untreated, this could lead to a number of health issues. From the foods we eat, to the environment we find ourselves in as well as the stress we encounter on a daily basis, all of these things can really weigh us down. In some cases, it actually contributes to our weight gain.

Ashtanga poses are designed with the philosophy of creating balance in the body. A clean body provides mental clarity and awareness, which has a significant influence on our overall lifestyle.

Alright, now that we have the basics covered, let's go straight into one of the poses that every beginner should be able to practice easily.

☐Sun Salutation

You will find this same pose in Vinyasa yoga but this one is longer and more in-depth. Begin the pose by standing upright on your mat. Keep your back straight and slowly lift your arms up, moving them over your head. Make sure that your palms are pressed firmly together.

From this pose, gently bend your torso forward, placing it against your thighs while you press both hands down onto the mat right beside your feet. Do this slowly as you will be stretching quite a bit to get your hands to reach the mat. If you are unable to do so during the first try, do not fret. You should be able to achieve this with constant practice.

Now, straighten your arms whilst making sure that your hands and feet remain still. Slowly, loft your head and gaze towards the ceiling. In this position, your body should be in the shape of a triangle. Hold this position for a few seconds before moving to the next one.

Lower your entire body onto the mat; you should be in a similar position to that of a push-up. From this pose, straighten your arms and try to lift your torso up, bending backwards gently. This pose is known as the upward-facing dog. Hold the pose for a bit, feeling the stretch, before lifting your bottom towards the ceiling just as you lower your torso once more. Point your head towards the floor whilst your legs and arms remain straight. In this pose, your body should be in an inverted V shape.

From this pose, slowly move both of your legs closer to your torso whilst placing your hands beside your feet on top of the mat. Allow your arms to bend a little and move your torso right against your thighs. Slowly begin to raise both your arms, along with your torso, upward until you are standing straight once more. Keep your palms together and stretch towards the sky as you do this. Once done, lower both arms and rest them at your sides.

These are the basic movements for Ashtanga yoga and are among the movements that many beginners should be able to do easily. Repeat the poses as much as you want to. You can add a bit more variety to it once you have managed to advance a bit more.

Benefits of Ashtanga Yoga:

People practice yoga for different reasons. Aside from helping you lose weight, it can also aid you in developing strength and boost your physical healing if you recently suffered an injury. To help you understand how Ashtanga yoga works on your body, here's a quick list of a few other benefits that it can provide you with:

☐ A lighter, more energized physical feeling

☐Stronger muscles and a greater range of motion for your joints

☐ Helps in improving your metabolism, digestion as well as your nutritional intake

☐Detoxifies the body

☐Restores any lost vitality

☐ Calms the mind and improves both memory as well as concentration

☐Improves the consciousness and quality of your breathing

☐ Can provide therapeutic relief for any muscle pain

Tips for Getting Started:

☐Try not to be intimidated. For beginners, the series of poses can seem daunting. However, do not let that scare you away from trying it. If you are doing it with a group, they will understand that you will not be as quick as the rest. This is the point of regular practice. For some people, it can take months before they are able to perform the poses smoothly. Just keep at it; practice at home too if you want to keep your flexibility up.

☐ Make small lifestyle changes. Starting Ashtanga yoga can also be the best time for you to jumpstart certain lifestyle changes that could help boost the practice's effects. Starting with your diet, you can reduce or completely remove meat from the daily menu and consume healthier substitute instead. It all depends on your preferences and what you are willing to do in order to maintain a healthy body. This is a great time for examining your current lifestyle choices and learning which ones truly benefit you, and which ones need to be changed.

☐ Breathe. When practicing any form of yoga, you will quickly learn that breathing is an important part of the process. Vinyasa, otherwise known as breath, links all of the postures associated with Ashtanga. There are certain poses wherein breathing seems almost impossible to do, such as the Halasana or Plow pose, but make sure that you do it. Just keep your breathing deep and steady. By breathing each time, you will be able to train and really allow yourself to go further into every pose you do.

Whether you choose to practice by yourself or with a group, always keep in mind that for this to help you with losing weight, it needs to be repeated as regularly as possible.

Warrior

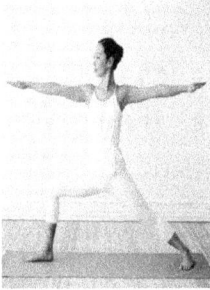

This is also known as the Dancing Warrior. It is done while standing and serves to stretch the waist. Reverse Warrior stretches strengthens the groins, legs, waist, hips and the sides of the torso It increases spine flexibility, inner thighs, chest and ankles. Additionally, it adds more strength to the arms, shoulders, and thighs. This pose increases blood circulation all over the body, thereby reducing tiredness and calming the mind. Regular practice of this pose builds stamina and helps relieve lower back pain. People with chronic joint injuries, hypertension and diarrhea should not practice this pose.

Stand with legs 3 to 4 feet apart, turning right foot out 90 degrees and left foot in slightly. Bring your hands to your hips and relax your shoulders, then extend arms out to the sides, palms down.

Bend right knee 90 degrees, keeping knee over ankle; gaze out over right hand. Stay for 1 minute.

Switch sides and repeat.

Mountain Pose

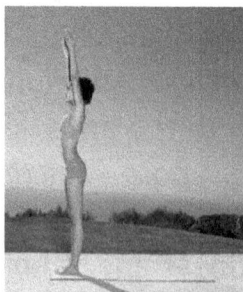

This pose is also known as Tadasana and is the premise of all the yoga poses done while standing. Tadasana when executed in the right way improves posture, tones abdominal muscles, and strengthens feet, thighs and ankles. It also calms the mind and the central nervous system thereby relieving stress and increasing concentration. Additionally, it helps in relieving sciatica and reduces the impacts of flat feet. Caution should be taken by persons suffering from hypertension, insomnia, balance issues and headaches.

Stand tall with feet together, shoulders relaxed, weight evenly distributed through your soles, arms at sides. Take a deep breath and raise your hands overhead, palms facing each other with arms straight. Reach up toward the sky with your fingertips.

Cobra

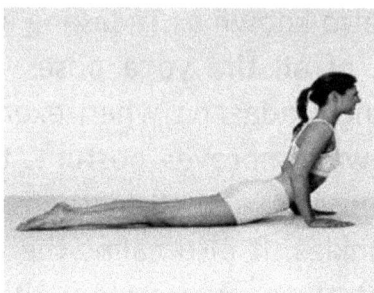

Lie facedown on the floor with thumbs directly under shoulders, legs extended with the tops of your feet on the floor. Tighten your pelvic floor, and tuck hips downward as you squeeze your glutes. Press shoulders down and away from ears.

Push through your thumbs and index fingers as you raise your chest toward the wall in front of you.

Relax and repeat.

Downward Dog

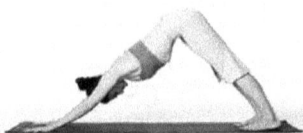

This is the most fundamental and popular pose in yoga. It is done while standing and bending to form the letter 'V'. When done consistently and in the right way, it deepens respiration, improves blood circulation, strengthens wrists, decreases anxiety, decreases tension headaches, elongates cervical spine and decreases back pain. This pose should be avoided by pregnant women in their third trimester, individual's suffering from carpal tunnel syndrome and those who experience sharp pain during practice.

Start on all fours with hands directly under shoulders, knees under hips. Walk hands a few inches forward and spread fingers wide, pressing palms into mat. Curl toes under and slowly press hips toward ceiling, bringing your body into an inverted V, pressing shoulders away from ears. Feet should be hip-width apart, knees slightly bent.

Hold for 3 full breaths.

Triangle Pose

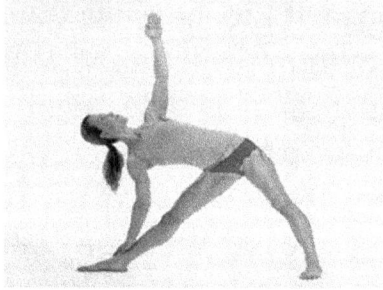

This is also known as Trikonasana and is executed while standing. This pose also requires the yogi to keep their eyes open in order to maintain body balance. This pose aids in strengthening the limbs and the chest, increases physical and mental equilibrium, opens up the hip, improves digestion, reduces stress, back pain, anxiety and sciatica and stretches all the body muscles. This is contraindicated to people suffering from hypertension, diarrhea, headaches and low blood pressure.

Extend arms out to sides, then bend over your right leg. Stand with feet about 3 feet apart, toes on your right foot turned out to 90 degrees, left foot to 45 degrees.

Allow your right hand to touch the floor or rest on your right leg below or above the knee, and extend the fingertips of your left hand toward the ceiling. Turn your gaze toward the ceiling, and hold for 5 breaths.

Stand and repeat on opposite side.

Tree Pose

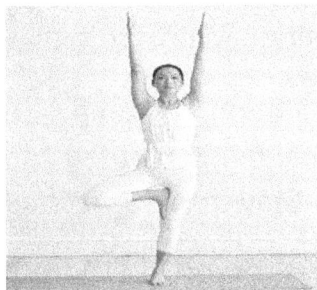

This pose is done balancing while standing. It makes a replica of the steady bearing of a tree. Eyes are kept open in order to maintain balance. It stretches your shoulders, inner thighs and groins, strengthens your feet and leg muscles, it builds balance, calm and relaxes your central nervous system as well as your mind and increases your mind and body awareness. The tree pose should be avoided by people suffering from insomnia, migraines hypotension and hypertension.

Stand with arms at sides. Shift weight onto left leg and place sole of right foot inside left thigh, keeping hips facing forward. Once balanced, bring hands in front of you in prayer position, palms together.

On an inhalation, extend arms over shoulders, palms separated and facing each other. Stay for 30 seconds. Lower and repeat on opposite side.

Make it easier: Bring your right foot to the inside of your left ankle, keeping your toes on the floor for balance. As you get stronger and develop better balance, move your foot to the inside of your left calf.

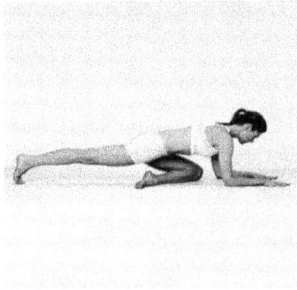

Pigeon Pose

Targets the piriformis (a deep gluteal muscle) Begin in a full push-up position, palms aligned under shoulders. Place left knee on the floor near shoulder with left heel by right hip. Lower down to forearms and bring right leg down with the top of the foot on the floor.

Keep chest lifted to the wall in front of you, gazing down. If you're more flexible, bring chest down to floor and extend arms in front of you.Pull navel in toward spine and tighten your pelvic-floor muscles; contract right side of glutes.

Curl right toes under while pressing ball of foot into the floor, pushing through your heel.

Bend knee to floor and release; do 5 reps total, then switch side's and repeat.

Bridge Pose

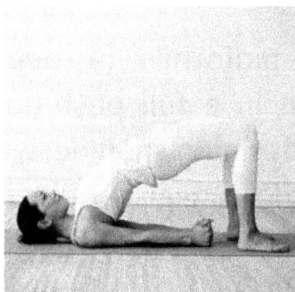

Stretches chest and thighs; extends spine. Lie on floor with knees bent and directly over heels.

Place arms at sides, palms down. Exhale, then press feet into floor as you lift hips. Clasp hands under lower back and press arms down, lifting hips until thighs are parallel to floor, bringing chest toward chin. Hold for 1 minute.

Make it easier: Place a stack of pillows underneath your tailbone.

Seated Twist

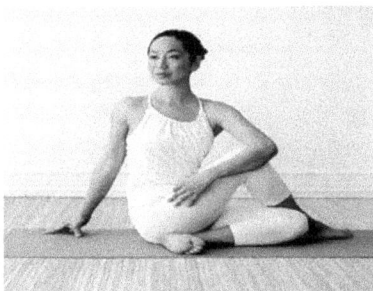

Stretches shoulders, hips, and back; increases circulation; tones abdomen; strengthens obliques. Sit on the floor with your legs extended. Cross right foot over outside of left thigh; bend left knee. Keep right knee pointed toward ceiling. Place left elbow to the outside of right knee and right hand on the floor behind you.

Twist right as far as you can, moving from your abdomen; keep both sides of your butt on the floor. Stay for 1 minute.

Switch sides and repeat.

Make it easier: Keep bottom leg straight and place both hands on raised knee. If your lower back rounds forward, sit on a folded blanket.

Crow Pose

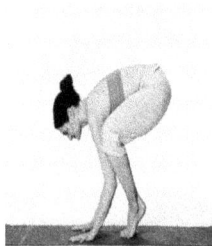

Get into downward dog position (palms pressed into mat, feet hip-width apart) and walk feet forward until knees touch your arms. Bend your elbows, lift heels off floor, and rest knees against the outside of your upper arms. Keep toes on floor, abs engaged and legs pressed against arms. Hold for 5 to 10 breaths.

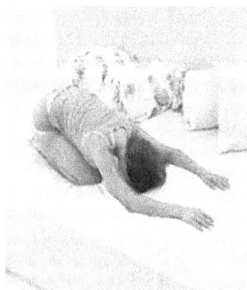

Child's Pose

Sit up comfortably on your heels. Roll your torso forward, bringing your forehead to rest on the bed in front of you. Lower your chest as close to your knees as you comfortably can, extending your arms in front of you.

Hold the pose and breathe.

Happiness, it is something that everyone seems to be searching for and many people are left without in life. The great thing about yoga is that it can help you find that happiness that you are looking for.

Of course, no one can be truly happy when they are in pain, using yoga to reduce the pain that you are dealing with on a regular basis is going to increase your happiness, but there is more to it than that.

If you have ever found yourself in a situation where you feel overwhelmed, tense or stressed, unable to calm down and unsure how to react, you probably know how important it is for you to take a few deep breaths to clear your mind.

Yoga will have the same effect on your mind, but it will not only help you in the instant that you are feeling overwhelmed

76

but it will help you from reaching that point. You will find that your unhealthy attitude, reactions and moods are shifted when you use meditation and yoga.

By using yoga, you will be less likely to suffer from depression, mood swings, anxiety, tension and fatigue. Not only that, but if you are already suffering from these issues, you will find that the symptoms begin to disappear when you begin practicing yoga on a regular basis.

Yoga will help to clear any energy blockages that are known as Sanskrit. When these are released, we are able to let our physical self and emotional self, flow more freely.

When you practice yoga you will also find that you are able to think more clearly. Think about the last time that something happened to upset you and you over reacted or reacted in a way that you regret. When you use Yoga, you are going to have fewer and fewer of those moments that you regret because your mind will be clear, you will be relaxed enough to not let tension or stress get to you and you will be able to take a step back, take a breath and look at the entire situation before reacting.

Yoga is also going to give you more energy. How many times have you found yourself wanting to get certain things done, planning to get them done and then at the end of the day finding that you have completed nothing? This happens to everyone, but if we are not careful, we can get stuck in a rut, this becomes a habit that is very hard to break. Often times, the reason for this is because you simply do not have the energy to do the things that you need to get done on a regular basis.

One thing that I have found over the years is that more and more people are suffering from fatigue and it is affecting their quality of life. There is no possible way to truly be happy when you are physically and mentally exhausted all of the time. Of course, it is very difficult to get a person to understand that they will have more energy after they begin practicing yoga.

On top of all of this, yoga will help you focus better which means that you will be more productive, of course bringing you more happiness. If you lose weight you will find that you feel a lot happier, by boosting your immunity, you will be healthier and happier.

Yoga will also help to reduce menstrual pain which is going to make plenty of women and girls much happier. It can also help to reduce migraines and help you sleep better.

Yoga brings happiness into your life because everything begins to fall into place. When you are not dealing with weight issues, health issues, sleep problems or stress, you will find that you are much happier. You will also find that yoga helps you to feel at peace in your mind. This means that instead of having racing thoughts you will be able to focus on one thought at a time. You will be able to solve one problem at a time without becoming overwhelmed and that will bring a lot of happiness into your life.

The fact is, all of these issues steal your happiness. By getting these issues under control you will be taking control of your happiness, taking it back and taking control of your life.

All of the exercises that I have given you in this book are going to help you reach a level of happiness in your life that you have never imagined was possible.

Balance is an essential part of yoga and will happen with ease as you begin to practice various poses. The more you become flexible and strong, the easier it will be to maintain your balance. There are a couple of poses that require you to be more balanced than you have been in the past or perhaps have been in these last few months. Virabhadrasana II is also the Warrior II pose. It asks you to be balanced between your feet to your head by using all parts of your body to maintain a perfect position. It is just one of many ways you can work on your center of gravity.

Step 12: Warrior II

Place your feet three to four feet apart. Start with the right foot, turning it slightly to be parallel to your body. With your left leg, you will have it bent at the knee and turned at a 90-degree angle. Your heel should be in line with the arch of your right foot. Your right leg will face forward slightly to be in line with your foot, but not bent. For your hips, turn them out or widen them, so that your upper body will still be parallel with your right leg. Keep your arms at shoulder height and outstretched. They should extend over your left knee and back past the unbent leg. Your head should turn to look over your left arm. Your chest will feel open and in line with your hips, while your spine will be straight from the hips up until the neck. Hold this pose for thirty seconds, at least three times. As you work on your balance, you can increase how long you hold the pose. You want to strengthen your legs and ankles while you are in this pose, but also maintain balance throughout your body. One of the best parts about Warrior II is how it helps your ankles. You are gaining strength in your ankle muscles because of how you turn your feet.

Step 13: Triangle

You should not attempt the triangle until you gain flexibility in your body. This means you need to bend without pain and be able to keep your legs straight, not bent at the knees. It is a great pose for working on your stamina and balance. You will start with your feet double the distance of your shoulders. Turn your right toes in slightly towards your body, while rotating your left leg open until you have your toes pointing to the side rather than in front of you. Keep your legs straight, and open your body from the hips through the chest, raising your arms to shoulder height, stretching them out through the fingertips. Once your arms are in the helicopter position, create a hinge with your hips by bending towards your left leg, placing your hand behind your leg. You do not need your palm flat, but to support your upper body with your fingertips. Your other arm will be in the air perfectly aligned with your shoulders. Turn your head to look up. Your legs will be your stand creating a triangle with the floor, while you bend at the waist. This is a great balance pose that also helps stretch your inner thighs and hamstrings.

Step 14: Tree

The tree is a simple balancing pose, more so than the two above. You will start in mountain pose, then raise one leg to bend at the knee. Your foot will turn inward towards your other leg's inner thigh, and you need to be as high on your leg as possible so that you are above the knee. Keep your foot flat, and your leg open, which also opens your hips. Lift your arms towards the ceiling, with your palms facing each other, and your fingers stretched out. Your head should balance with your spine. You are balancing on one foot. Change the position after a count of eight, repeat at least three times for each leg and build on this time as you get better at the position.

Step 15: Half Moon

Being with triangle pose for balance. Your front knee is bent in triangle pose; however, for Half Moon pose you are going to straighten it, while you raise the back foot off the mat. You are using your same hand to keep the balance and support you, as you lift your other leg to be in line with your spine. Your chest and head will be open towards the ceiling. The challenge is to keep the pose while balancing on one hand and leg. It requires concentration, as well as balance. This is a fantastic exercise to help you with anxiety if you are feeling anxious about anything in your mind. The focus it takes to remain in balance keeps your mind occupied on the pose alone versus the things that are stressing you.

CHAPTER 12: TIPS FOR USING MEDITATION WITH YOGA

What mostly differentiates yoga from other forms of exercise is its meditation aspect. Yoga meditation is an old Indian tradition that allows one to tap into all his senses and potentialities. The word "yoga" comes from the Sanskrit word "yuj," which is the origin of the English word "yoke." The word connotes as binding, or a union. In the yoga tradition, this suggests that all your divided pieces will become one, and you yourself will become one with the universe.

In yoga, you must clear your mind in order to be open to the world. It is often our close-mindedness that makes us miss the answers to our deepest questions.

Yoga meditation is usually facilitated with chants. These are sacred prayers that ancient practitioners have handed down to us through oral tradition.

The most common chant in yoga is "Aum" pronounced as "Om." The ancient Indian people believed that this primordial sound captures the entire universe. Myth has it that the Architect pronounced the syllable so perfectly that it created everything.

The   chant "Lokahsamasthasukhinobhavantu" is said to invoke wholeness with the world and a sense of wellness. It can be translated to mean "May all beings be happy and free." It takes your focus away from yourself and recognizes that the happiness of others is also your own.

"Om manipadme hum" are syllables that symbolize the body, speech and mind of the practitioner and of Buddha; enlightenment ("mani" means jewel); wisdom ("padme" means lotus). In Tibetan Buddhism, it is thought to be the most beneficial chant and is found carved in religious artifacts.

For those who are wary of chanting ancient prayers, you can just think of chants as a way to regulate your breath. The vibrations that the sounds form are also calming, similar to the effect of a meditation bell or gong.

The perfect pose for meditation is "Padmasana" or The Lotus, which is, in essence, a cross-legged sitting position. A "half lotus" is done with one foot resting on top of the opposite leg's thigh. A "full lotus" is achieved with both feet resting on their opposite thighs. You can rest your hands on top of your knees or place them in prayer position with palms together in the center of your chest. You can also place your fingers in yoga mudra position with your thumb touching your index finger and the rest of your fingers outstretched. Set the back of your hands on top of your knees.

Pranayama is about aligning the conscious mind with the regulation of the life force. In other words, it is about using your conscious mind to perform an otherwise unconscious act – breathing. This does two things. The first is the obvious physiological changes that come from altering the depth of breathing and the frequency. Being attached to a pulse-oxygen monitor will show an increase in oxygen saturation. The increase in these levels allows the body to expel toxins that are stored, rejuvenate the cells, and increase the flow of energy.

The second benefit of this is psychological. The attachment of psyche to breathing focuses the mind on its rhythmic wave. It's like starring at a hypnotist's pendulum. The ebb and flow of breathing are hypnotic and can aid in the resetting of the mind. That, in its self, is a powerful way to rejuvenate.

Four breathing techniques come under the heading of Pranayama. These techniques allow you to vary the frequency and amplitude of your breathing. The key to optimizing one's benefit from breathing is to vary the sequence and to focus on the actual act. The central theme of the breathing exercises, you will notice, are the acts that run parallel with the breathing. All of them are designed to change something that otherwise is regular and boring.

Cooling Breath

The body generates a lot of heat in the normal process of daily activity. To dissipate that heat, the body uses several mechanisms. One of them is perspiration. When the moisture on the skin is heated by the temperature of the body, it is energized. When it evaporates, it takes the energy that was transferred from the skin. That process cools the body down. When one urinates, it takes the heat found in the contents of the bladder and releases it. That is also cooling. The third way is by breathing. When we breathe, large volumes of blood, carrying gasses and heat enter the lungs to deposit their gasses, and in the process transfer the heat that they have picked up during their journey around the body. This heat is transferred to the lungs much like the coolant in the engine moves to the radiator in a car. As the carbon dioxide transfers to the lungs, it carries heat with it and it expels that heat with the characteristic warm breath that exists our mouth and nostrils. In return, the ambient air brings with it cooler temperature and transfers that temperature to the blood as it goes around the body.

When we exert energy, our natural metabolic process generates heat as a byproduct. That heat, whether we feel it or otherwise, remains trapped inside. That excess heat reduces the efficacy of the chemical reactions in some cases and accelerates it in other cases. This dual effect throws the natural rhythm and process into chaos. Reduced efficacy of the chemical process results in degraded health.

To conduct this exercise, sit up straight. Be comfortable without stretching or extending your chest muscles. Once you attain a comfortable posture, tilt your nose slightly above the horizon. Open your mouth and shape it as though you are about to say a pronounced letter 'O.' However, don't make any sound. Roll your tongue back and let the tip touch the roof of your mouth. This will cause the underside of your tongue to face the incoming air as you inhale with your mouth.

In Sanskrit, this is called Sitali Pranayama.

Forced Exhale

As we go about our daily activities, it is common to reduce ourselves to shallow breathing. This is done inadvertently. That has side effects in the short and long-term. Extended periods of shallow breathing reduces the lung's capacity and raises the acidity of the systems. Acidity in the body leads to poor health. The blood is best maintained at a slightly elevated pH – 7.2 which indicates a balance that is tipped lightly towards alkali.

This exercise should be done for at least ten minutes in the day, every day. It is also beneficial to do this exercise more than once for those who have sedentary lifestyles. For those who sit in the office every day and do not have to move, the need to breathe heavily is diminished. This exercise will rectify that and reduce pH levels.

To do this, sit up straight with your nose pointed over the horizon. Push your chest slightly forward and your shoulders slightly to the rear. Focus on your natural breathing until you find the subconscious rhythm – the rate and depth that your body is doing on its own. Keep a note of the time it takes to inhale and exhale.

Maintain that span of the inhalation cycle, but take in a deeper breath. For instance, if it takes one second for you to complete an inhalation cycle, use that same time to take a deeper breath. This means you will be inhaling a little deeper, at a faster pace. To exhale, the time is doubled. The exhalation is done by pushing your diaphragm to evacuate the air, but at the same time constricting the escape at the throat. This blockage will create pressure in the chest while the volume of air is slowly allowed to escape. If you can't hold it in your throat, purse your lips to control the exit of air. Do this for about ten minutes at a time.

The common mistake in doing this is the excess exhalation that eventually reduces the amount of carbon dioxide in the lungs. To prevent this, or to reduce the feeling of discomfort, take a deep breath and hold the air in. This will return the saturation of CO_2 to normal levels. At that point, you can continue with your exercise.

In Sanskrit, this is called Ujjayi Pranayama.

Explosive Exhaling

In a move that exaggerates the forced exhale, this explosive exhale is designed to clear the passages. Our breathing passages can get blocked with mucus and pockets of air that develop. In the normal course of breathing the force of incoming and outgoing air is insufficient to clear these pockets of liquid and gas. It's like a faint blow of a birthday candle that refuses to extinguish. To extinguish the flame, you have to blow at it with some vigor. That's what this explosive hailing is designed to do, except you are not blowing out your birthday candle, your unseating pockets of liquid and air that may be stuck in your passages.

To do this, sit back in a comfortable posture. The goal is to straighten your spine and tilt your head back. This has the effect of reducing the stresses on your back muscles. It also allows you to sit straight for a longer period. Inhale deeply and hold your breath until the count of three. One, one thousand, two one thousand, three one thousand. The push all the air out in one explosive push. This is preferably done through the nose. It is, however, a reality that those with sinus blockages would not be able to do this all through their nose. If you are one of those with permanent sinus blockage, then work your way up to how rapidly you can exhale. The key is that it should be done via the nostrils and not the mouth. Part of the reason nasal blockages in the sinus occur is that the blockages that should have been cleared were allowed to remain and that gradually resulted in permanent constriction of the passages.

Explosive exhaling can be tiring as it is working the diaphragm that is normally not used in this way. Doing it 30 times a day can be exhausting. If so, start with half the amount and work your way up to it. There are two common issues with explosive exhaling. We've already looked at one – the sinus blockages. The second is when one does the act too rapidly and too deeply. It will result in too much carbon dioxide being exhaled and you could feel light-headed. The remedy for this is the same as the last exercise that resulted in the same problem. Take a deep breath and hold it until you feel better, then exhale slowly. Do it until you feel you can inhale and exhale normally.

This exercise in Sanskrit is called Kapalabhati Pranayama.

Nostril Exercise

The last of the four breathing exercises is to lie down flat without the benefit of a pillow to elevate your head. If you find this uncomfortable, you can use a flat pillow to raise your head slightly but not more. Use your dominant hand to alternate the closing of your nostrils. Raise your dominant hand to your nose. Take a deep breath and exhale, and do it three times. Once you have cleared your lungs for the last time, press your right nostril with your dominant hand and inhale with the open nostril until your belly is fully extended. Control the volume of air intake with the movement of your belly rather than your chest.

Once you reach the comfortable peak of inhalation, hold your breath while you switch nostrils, and exhale from your right nostril. When you have finished exhaling, that will mark half a cycle. Now inhale from the same nostril you just exhaled from, keeping the other nostril shut with your finger. Once the lungs are full, hold your breath. Now switch nostrils and exhale with the nostril that you just opened up. This is one full cycle.

In this one full cycle, you have inhaled once, and exhaled once in one nostril, and done the same on the other. Do at least ten full cycles, then observe the way your body and mind feel. You will notice a perceptible difference in mood, concentration, and quality of energy.

You do not need to do this daily although nothing is stopping you from doing it. You will find the most benefit if you do this during times when you can't fall asleep or feel anxious. If your mind starts to wander, this technique helps to bring it back to earth and helps with anxiety.

Anxiety is an energy of the mind that places it in chaos. Breathing in this way allows the mind to relax, whereupon it can be rationalized and returned to positive thinking.

In Sanskrit, this is called Nadhi Sodana.

We began this book stating the point that Yoga is the convergence of multiple dimensions of existence. We saw pose and motion, and we saw thoughts to promote and actions to avoid. Now we have just witnessed the importance of breathing. If nothing else, the adoption of healthy breathing habits is paramount to the development of a peaceful and fulfilled life. The brain, our seat of consciousness and cognitive ability, is fueled by the metabolic process that is dependent on the proper balance of oxygen and carbon dioxide. Lethargy, reduced focus, depression, anxiety, poor motivation are all side effects of poor breathing habits.

The breathing techniques described here provide a full spectrum of exercises to promote smooth and balanced gaseous exchange.

On their own, they make a significant impact. However, when combined with the Asanas, the body undergoes a transformation that is visible and recognizable. There is a better quality of energy and a reduced need for food. Proper Yoga techniques – not just the poses and posture, but the combined limbs of Yoga, have the effect of increasing the absorption of nutrients and the extraction of energy from the food that is consumed.

One gains excess weight because there is a lowered intake of nutrients and poor breathing habits. Poor breathing habits reduce the metabolic process. It is like a poorly calibrated fuel injection system. When there is insufficient oxygen entering the mix, the fuel does not burn well and the driver instinctively gives it more gas. Consumption goes through the roof, but there is still no power. The same goes for the human metabolic engine. Reduced oxygen results in poor energy output and that tends to make the person eat more. To eat something when feeling low is a natural instinct. Interpreting the condition as needing fuel is reactionary. That increased intake is stored as fat. Weight gain compounds the problem.

Once breathing habits are fixed, and the metabolic engine is running at optimum levels, the body burns up what it needs and doesn't feel sluggish or need more food to do the same level of work.

CHAPTER 14: WHERE CAN I LEARN YOGA AND WHAT DO I NEED?

In the course of this book, I have talked about how yoga is beneficial for many aspects of your life. However, you might be wondering how you can become involved with yoga. Well, there are many different answers to this question, so I thought that I would cover some of the many ways you can become involved in yoga depending on your schedule and preferences. Since not every person likes to do the same things and yoga is a popular form of exercise, there are many ways you can become involved in making it a part of your life.

Getting prepared to do yoga requires minimal materials. All you really need is a mat and a clear space to work in. If you're using a video, then a television and disc player are necessary as well. Find clothing that is suitable for physical activity. However, make sure that you're comfortable in your clothing, otherwise it might affect your focus on the yoga poses.

If you like soothing music while performing yoga, you might want to have classical or nature music playing at a low volume. Make your surroundings as comfortable and soothing as possible before you begin.

The next step in starting a yoga routine is to find out how you would like to do your routine. This can be anywhere from a yoga studio to your backyard. Find a place that feels peaceful and tranquil to you and make that space your yoga space. The number one thing to remember is that you need to feel comfortable with your surroundings in order for yoga to be beneficial to you.

When considering how you would like to learn yoga, think about what you would prefer for your setting and instructional method. Are you the type of person who feels comfortable in a public setting, or do you prefer to exercise in the privacy of your own home? Think about what you like when reading this chapter and try a couple of the ways that sound good to you.

Yoga Classes

If you have ever come across an advertisement for a gym, then you have probably noticed that many gyms offer some form of a yoga class. There are even studios that are devoted to nothing but yoga. If you're a social person and like to take classes, then finding a yoga class in your area might be a great solution for you. Also, if you like to be coached and told what to do and when, an instructor that can lead you and guide you is necessary. Some people need to know that they're performing the moves correctly and the only way to make sure of this is to have someone watch you and tell you what you're doing wrong.

By taking a class, you are setting aside a specific time in your schedule for your personal health. A class offers you a structure and guidance that you may not get if you practice alone. An instructor is also a good source of coaching and information that can help you get the most out of your yoga experience. The great part about some gyms and studios is that they offer a free class to start. This will give you an idea of whether or not a yoga class is right for you.

Instructional Videos

You can see them in almost any department store that has a sports section. Exercise videos. Amongst them, a great number of them are devoted to yoga. Since there is a wide variety of yoga videos on the market, this is another way that you can get guidance on how to perform yoga. Even though you won't have a live instructor, a good instructional video will help you know how to complete the poses and when to breathe while performing them.

Videos are a great way for someone who has a sporadic schedule to be able to get some time to exercise in. It is easy to put in and follow whenever you have a free moment. However, this might be a problem for some who need to plan their routines ahead of schedule. It is easy to put that video aside just because you don't feel like doing it. Also, there are many not so great videos out there. Take some time and find out which ones are recommended by others before investing in a yoga instructional video.

Video Gaming Systems

Almost every gaming platform out there offers games that are devoted to fitness. Yoga is one of the most popular fitness games out there. The Wii gaming system offers you the opportunity to do yoga with the aid of a balance board and a motion detector. When you're off balance, the board records it for you to see. This is a great way to be able to work out and have the guidance to correct your body movements if needed. The program will also guide you on when to breathe and help you to remember to keep your muscles steady.

Like instructional videos, doing yoga with a video game is a less structured way to do a workout. You can do it on your own schedule, but you really have no advice on which poses will work for you personally. By knowing which poses affect which parts of the body, you can find the poses that might suit you the best. However, the convenience of being able to work out in your own home on your own schedule is enticing to many.

Books and Magazines

The techniques of yoga and how to practice it is also readily available in books. These books offer pictures that will help you see how the poses are executed and give you written directions on how to do the pose. This is great for those who have to see something in order to understand it.

There are also magazines out there that highlight the practice of yoga. Fitness magazines often run articles on yoga and the different poses that will help you achieve results. You can also find magazines that are strictly devoted to yoga and leading a yoga lifestyle. By getting updated advice and articles, you are keeping yourself prepared for finding methods that will work best for you.

While books and magazines might need to be combined with other methods to make them more effective, they offer great insights and advice from people who practice yoga on a regular basis. They also offer tips for people who might not pick up on yoga as quickly as others. Try looking through a book or a magazine while visiting a bookstore and see if it offers any advice that will benefit you.

Internet

Like anything else, there are many resources on the internet that will help you find the right poses and the correct execution of the poses. Explore some of the popular websites and find out which poses are good for you and how to do them. There are also videos on YouTube and other websites that offer direction on how to perform yoga. However, you need to be careful about the reliability of the information you find on the internet. Like instructional videos, there are many poor yoga videos posted on the internet. Look at the user ratings before trying them out because they will be a good guide on how well it worked for others.

No matter what you prefer, there are many solutions to how to get your yoga instruction. Find which one will work out the best for you and make it a routine to perform your yoga on regular basis. It will help with your physical and mental health!

CHAPTER 15: PRANAYAMA

Pranayama is derived from the two Sanskrit words 'prana', which means vital energy and 'ayama' which means control. Therefore literally interpreted pranayama means control of your vital energy. However, it is more generally interpreted and understood as control of the breath, which in yoga philosophy is often associated or interpreted with 'vital energy' and the life force.

Techniques used in pranayama work on the basis that the breathing can be controlled to follow certain rhythms, which can relax or focus the body and mind. Furthermore, by learning to breathe efficiently, pranayama also claims you can improve your energy levels and overall vitality.

To be more precise, pranayama is believed not only to contribute to weight loss, but help purify the blood, remove toxins, improve clarity and concentration, increase our pain threshold and lower experiences of pain as well as make us feel peaceful and calm. It is quite the list of benefits!

Depending on your source material, there may be dozens of different pranayama techniques. Some types of yoga also associate prana with energy and associate them with specific regions in the body, similar in principle to chakras. To yogi's mental energy or emotion are just a type of prana, but all these different kinds of prana originate from the breath.

Moreover the breath also influences how this prana is exchanged in the body. Fast, rapid breathing results in quick short bursts of energy, whilst slow rhythmic breathing creates steady, continuous energy flows. These different energy flows in turn influence our state of mind, with slower types of breathing producing relaxed and stable mental states.

Similarly, over time these types of breathing and energy flows influence the body. Short, constricted breathing damages the body over time and may contribute to sickness and fatigue. Conversely, deep, efficient breathing strengthens the body with energy, making you resistant and durable. Eventually these bodily changes, originating from the breath, are thought to influence our personality. Disturbed breathing leads to an unsettled mind; calm breathing leads to a calm mind.

In ancient texts, prana was believed to channel and coalesce in small points in the body called nadis, with some texts suggesting that there are up to 72,000 nadis in the body. In modern times the flow of prana through the body has become associated with the nervous system and the flow of energy from the brain and spinal cord into all the smaller branches of nerves throughout the body.

The purpose of pranayama is to change the breathing to originate from the navel and the base of the spine, rather than the nostrils of chest. Although you do not need to believe in the spiritual systems that the ancient yogis believed, it is thought that breathing in such a way will open the root chakra, which in turn can contribute and lead to higher spiritual awakening.

On the same vein, pranayama is considered to be part of Raja yoga, or royal yoga, which concerns the more esoteric and spiritual aspects of yoga. Many westerners have adopted these practices to lower stress, combat depression and increase their overall satisfaction with life.

The most basic stage of pranayama is to focus upon the breath. This type of breathing meditation is a staple of many religious and spiritual practices in the East. By continually focusing on the breath, the mind and concentration is refined and improved, which can lead to deeper and more advanced states of meditation.

To start, sit in a comfortable position in a room free from distractions. It is preferable if this is a room where you do not usually spend a large amount of your time, so it is free from your usual mental associations and habits. Ideally you would sit in the half-lotus position or perfect pose, where one foot rests on the thigh of the opposite leg. However, if this is too strenuous and uncomfortable for you, kneeling or sitting in other positions is sufficient.

Your aim when focusing upon the breath is to develop diaphragmatic breathing. The diaphragm is a muscle below the lungs which contracts and expands as you breathe. Deeper breathing is associated with a greater level of movement within the diaphragm, whereas shallow breathing is associated with the chest and shoulders.

According to yogis there are three types of breathing, diaphragmic breathing with originates around the belly button, thoracic breathing (mid-chest) and clavicular breathing (upper chest). Often these different types of breathing are simplified as deep, moderate and shallow breathing respectively.

Deep breathing is thought to be the most efficient. Shallow breathing can occur during exercise, but also if the breathing is damaged through smoking or asthma. Moderate breathing tends to be the typical mode of breathing for most people. Based upon the previous understanding that breathing affects our overall mood, bodily health and personality, it can be concluded that we can in a sense, improve yourself simply by learning to breathe deeply.

To practice deep breathing, simply breathe through your nose, but try to breathe slowly. It is thought we breathe around 15-20 times per minute. According to pranayama experts, it is best if you can breathe less than this.

Whilst you breathe rest your hand against your belly (diaphragm). When you inhale your diaphragm should be forced out and it should contract when you exhale. If you are struggle to breathe this deeply, than try to empty your lungs of air first. Exhale to the maximum extent possible and wait for a few seconds to breathe inwards again – your next breathe will be much deeper and should originate from the belly.

In particular, when you are trying to breathe slower, your aim should be specifically to inhale slower. It is thought that allowing the air to fill and stay within your lungs longer, your increase the amount of oxygen your body intakes and boost metabolic activity.

A more advanced pranayama technique involves placing a weight on the belly whilst you lay down and breathe. This is intended to strengthen the diaphragm and extend all the benefits of the basic pranayama even further.

Additionally, it is thought that pausing the breath between inhalation and exhalation can be beneficial. Try to give a small 1-2 second pause between your inhalation and exhalation, but do not make yourself light-headed if this feels too uncomfortable.

For a beginner, that is all you need to do. It sounds simple, but once you have tried to control your breathing for an extended period of time, you should notice it is in fact rather hard. The mind has a natural tendency to wander and deep stress and anxieties come forward. If this happens to you, try to persist.

Stress is naturally uncomfortable and your mind has a natural habit to flee and distract itself. Don't allow this! Simply feel your stress or anxiety in all its subtle complexity and overwhelming power. Although it may take time, as you continue to breathe deeply, these feelings will subside and diminish. You don't conquer stress this way; you allow it flow and dissipate, and ultimately become peaceful and tranquil.

CHAPTER 16: YOGA MUDRAS POSES

Mudras are described as hand positions. Each area of the hand has a reflex reaction in a specific part of the brain. A Mudra locks and guides energy flow and reflexes to the brain.

Gyan MudraGyan Mudra

Place together the tips of the index finger and thumb . The index finger represents the planet Jupiter and Jupiter represents knowledge and expansion. The pose above is one of the most commonly used Mudras.

Shuni Mudra

Place together the tips of the middle finger and thumb. The middle finger is associated with Saturn. The planet Saturn represents patience
, discernment, and the law of karma. This means one should be courageous and responsible.

118

Surya Ravi Mudra

Place together the tips of the ring finger and thumb. The ring finger is associated with the sun or Uranus. The Sun represents energy, health, and sexuality. Uranus represents the nervous system, strength, intuition, and change. continue

Buddhi Mudra

Place together the tip of the pinky and thumb. The pinky finger it is associated with Mercury. Mercury represents quickness, and the power of communication.

Venus Lock

The name Venus Lock is derived from the connection between the negative and positive side of the Venus mounds. These are located on each hand and are the fleshy areas at the base of the thumb (which represents ego).

Prayer Mudra

This mudra neutralizes the positive (male) and negative (female) side of the body. This position is always done before starting a Yoga class. By pressing the palms of the hands together firmly, we connect the two hemispheres of the brain, and bringing them into balance. continue

Bear Grip

This Mudra is used to stimulate the heart and to intensify concentration.

Hands In Lap

This Mudra it is commonly used for meditation.

Yoga Mudras Practice For Daily Life

Mudras are the sign language of yoga, often referred to as energetic 'seals' as they can alter our attitude and perceptions, while deepening awareness and concentration. They're just as important as the chaturanga or the backbend because like all asanas, mudras remind us that happiness comes from within a very deep place inside ourselves...and it's our job to call it up.

! Here are five mudras that will change your inner/outer world as fast as you do them.

1. Abaya Mudra — Be Fearless. Call On Courage. DO YOU!

In this mudra, raise your right hand to shoulder height with your fingers extended and palm turned outward. Looks like you're swearing under oath. It's the, 'I-swear-to-tell-the-truth-the-whole-truth-and-nothing-but-the-truth-so-help-me-God" mudra.

It's not your business what other people think of you. Stand in the middle of your fear with courage or have the fear and do it anyway.

2. Ganesh — Meet The Remover Of Obstacles.

In this mudra, clasp your hands in front of your heart and tug 100 miles an hour on the exhale and relax on the inhale. Do this three times on each side, sit and feel the effects.

Often Ganesh puts apparent obstacles in our way so that we can see them and have the opportunity to do the work of removing them, stretching us to grow and change.

3. Shiva Shakti — Engage Your Energy.

In this mudra, place your right hand with thumb extended upward, on top of your left open hand. Position hands near your belly with elbows pointing wide. Free breathing or pump it up, literally!

Ready to give your energy a massive boost and blast into new positive life enhancing habits, you can even add some breath of fire or kappalabhati breathing into this, moving any stuck (old) energy from your lower centers and chakras to move upward. This is your natural Prozac.

4. Lotus Mudra — Open Your Heart To All Situations & Beings.

In this mudra, your hands meet in the front of the heart, palms open forming a lotus with thumbs and pinkie fingers touching. Out of the mud comes the most beautiful flower, this is the story of our transformation each and every day. With daily practice we can stay open and loving.

5. Anjali Mudra — Practice Gratitude.

In this mudra, fold your hands into a prayer at your heart, the lotus hands merge together into a Namaste. Our hands become instruments for healing our mind and body and connecting us in this sacred way to our highest self!

Gratitude. Every breath is a blessing, every breath is a second change. Count your blessings loves! We have so much to be grateful for. Focus on what you have. My two favorite words: THANK YOU! Say them as much as you can.

If you're new to the practice of mudras I recommend a 40-day sadhana, or practice, to change your world. Habits can be made holy and joyful practices. Practice your mudra each and every day around the same time and repeat them with awareness on your breathing. You will feel your prana, force of life change, shift.

Try all of them, and if you're drawn to one mudra in particular, stay with that one and repeat it daily for 40 days. Start your morning with your mudra and see where it shows and flows in the rest of your day.

Using our hands in this powerful way is the ultimate high-five. It's my high five to you, family.

Yoga Mudras Practice For WEight Loss

Surya Mudra

Method : Fold the ring finger holding it from thumb which has to press down keeping the other fingers straight and place the hands on the knees and palms facing the sky forms Surya Mudra. Do this for 20 to 30 minutes followed by Prana Mudra for 10 minutes. Surya Mudra can be practised while walking also. It can be practiced in other times as well.

Benefits:

1) increases heat in the body as sun is the giver of energy.

2) increase of heat dissolves the fat stored in body cells

3) improves digestion & reduces obesity due to excess fat

4) all problems of thyroid gland reduces or eliminated

5) sometime due to thyroid , menses abnormalities are caused, which reduces.

6) decreases mental heaviness

7) reduces chlorostral , constipation

8) helpful in diabetes, TB, ASTHAMA

9) balances body.

Earth element will be reduced by doing this. Cholesterol accummulated in the body will vanish thereby reducing the unnecessary weight. Problem of phlegm, sinusitis, cold, pneumonia, TB, asthma can be cured. Do this mudra followed by Linga Mudra for 7 to 8 minutes for better results. Digestion will improve. You will live in enthusiasm. Efficiency in the working of thyroid gland will increase.

Caution : Persons with weakness should NOT do this mudra. If above problems are found, do this mudra for a minute, see the result, if no difficulty is experienced, then practise this, that too for a little time only.

Linga Mudra

Method : Interlock fingers of both hands keeping one thumb in erect position and other thumb coming round the first one as shown in the figure. Do this for 5 to 6 minutes.

Benefits: Since many acupressure points are pressed simultaneously, efficiency of heart, thyroid gland, lever, neck will increase. If you do this during winter, body will get heated up in a few minutes. Diseases like cough, cold, sinus, asthma, pneumonia, TB will be cured. Diseases that recur during weather change will vanish. Cholesterol and proteins are melted which help in decreasing body weight.

Do this followed by Surya Mudra to control increasing body weight. Solar plexus will come to its original place and digestion will be normal. For details of solar plexus, see page No.73.

Attention : By doing Linga Mudra, body gets heated up. Hence please drink sufficient water. And also take fruit juice, milk, buttermilk, lemon sharabath, etc. to avoid ill-effects of this mudra.

Caution: People suffering from Pitha (Bile) related problems should NOT do this mudra. Please note that those who suffer from acidity, giddiness, ulcer don't do this. When there is cold, phlegm, do this for 2 minutes only and stop immediately after the problem is averted.

A mudra believed to specifically help with weight loss is called Surya Mudra. Many believe that it can help cure obesity. It is said to control hunger and temptation for food and change the metabolism so that it is easy to lose weight and maintain a healthy weight balance. Another mudra, Prithvi Mudra is said to reduce cholesterol in the body while helping to reduce weight.

Effects

The yoga mudras are utilized to seal the practitioner's intended wish, desire or thought focused upon in meditation. For the purposes of weight loss you may also use the mudras of health, vitality and energy to make changes to your metabolism and digestion of food.

Benefits

It is believed that practicing these mudras regularly can yield health benefits. Yogic philosophy assigns specific internal organs to each of the fingers, and so holds that using mudras will correspond to enhanced function of internal organs. Many are said to cure mental heaviness, reduce body fat, normalize blood pressure and even strengthen the heart.

CHAPTER 17: MASSAGE THOSE FEET!

Self-Massage

Most people love a good foot massage. It can feel so amazing to massage your feet. It's good for the feet and also stimulates other parts of the body at the same time. You have all of these acupressure points in your foot that connect to other parts of the body. So, a foot massage is like a massage for other parts of the body at the same time. Bonus!

Massaging your feet also helps to loosen the muscles and connective tissue in your feet. Some of those aches in your feet are caused by tight muscles or connective tissue. Taking a few minutes to rub your feet can bring a little relief to them.

There's really no perfect way to massage your feet. So, don't worry about doing it wrong. It can be nice to start with a favorite lotion or some massage oil in your hands. Then begin to rub your feet. Start with some lighter strokes and then, if it feels right, you can focus on any tight spots that you feel. You'll quickly get to know your feet this way. Maybe there's one spot that's always sore. If that is happening, then spend a little extra time on that spot. Be firm but gentle. Don't forget the top of the foot or the heel and ankle.

Spread Those Toes!

It's also really nice to place a finger in between each toe. Try to work a finger in between each toe all at the same time.

While this isn't really a massage, after spending all day smooshed into shoes that are really constricting, this will feel really good. Spread out your toes. Give your feet the space that they crave. If you're lucky enough to walk barefoot often, then your feet will naturally spread out a bit. By putting a finger between each toe, you're just helping those toes find a naturally spacious experience. Do it often enough and your feet will start to feel

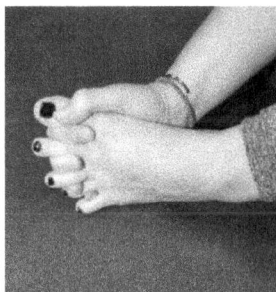

better!

Another simple idea is to simply spread your toes apart. In the pictures below, you can see a foot with the toes as they normally are. The second picture is the toes spread apart. At first, this might be difficult to do, but the more you practice simply putting a little space between the toes, the easier it will be.

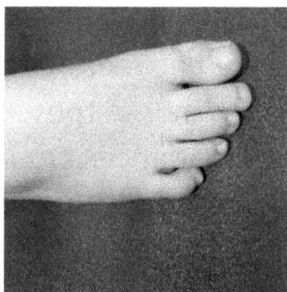

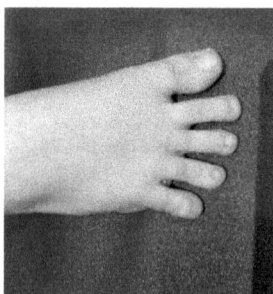

Normal foot with toes together.

Foot with toes spread apart.

Use a Massage Ball

Try a Massage Ball. I have several small massage balls. They are so helpful when you want to massage your feet. I'll be honest. If you've got tight/sore spots, then this might be a bit more painful than if you massage your own feet. However, these massage balls do a terrific job of getting deeper into the tissue of the foot than you would with your own fingers.

How do you use a massage ball? Well, there are multiple ways. You can use your hand to move the ball around your foot and enjoy the way it feels. You can also take the ball and place it under your foot. Then, using a little of your body weight for extra pressure, you can begin to move your foot around on the ball. Again, this might hurt a bit because you're using extra pressure to go deeper into the tissue of the foot. So, judge the pressure based on how deep you want to go. Remember less is often more! In this case that might mean that you use just a little of your body weight and that will be enough. Practice kindness to yourself. Don't do too much too fast. I want you to be able to walk comfortably after this foot massage.

Try a foot bath A great way to relieve tired, stressed or sore feet is a foot bath. Fill a small tub with warm water and add in Epsom salts. You can also add in your favorite essential oil for added benefit. The Epsom salts will help to relieve soreness and swelling in the feet. They will help reduce your overall stress level. They'll also give you some extra magnesium and that magnesium will speed your recovery from standing on those feet all day long. It might even help you sleep better. There are so many benefits to using Epsom salt in your foot bath.

The essential oils can help your feet even more. I like a little lavender oil in mine. The lavender that I like helps to reduce inflammation and stress. It also helps to calm my mind and body at the same time.

Eucalyptus Oil also is a good choice. It can provide a cooling effect for your muscles as well as reduce pain and inflammation.

Peppermint Oil can revive tired feet.

Marjoram Oil can calm and soothes your muscles.

There are a lot of good options when it comes to essential oils. It might be that some days one oil is just what you need and other days, you need something else. Experiment and find the oils that work for you.

PracticeMindfulness

How often do you pay attention to your feet? Usually we notice our feet when they hurt but ignore them the rest of the time. What if you practiced a little mindfulness around your feet? Whenever you can, go barefoot and just notice what it feels like to walk around barefoot. Notice what it feels like to place your feet on the ground. Notice any sensations that move up your body from your feet. Notice if you have a preference for walking on one surface over another. Just begin to notice what happens when your feet touch the ground.

You can also practice mindfulness when you have shoes on. How do your feet feel in your shoes? Do your shoes encourage your foot to spread out a bit or are your shoes making your feet feel cramped? Do you need new shoes to make your feet feel better? Again, notice how it feels to take a step in your shoes. Notice if your shoes are making your feet feel energized or if they are making you feel tired. Notice if the rest of your body feels good while in your shoes or if your shoes are leading you to not feel good throughout the day. Also, notice if you're placing style over function.

I won't tell you that you have to go and buy shoes that are ugly, but make your feet feel great. However, I will ask that you try mindfulness in your shoes. Be aware of how your feet and the rest of your body feel while you're wearing your shoes. Maybe you want to stick with the pretty but uncomfortable shoes. That's okay. You can do that. Just be aware of how you feel while you wear those shoes.

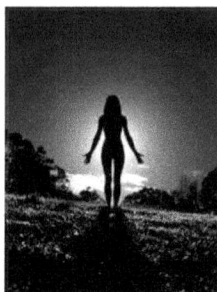

This section introduces some of the basic yoga postures starting from a standing position. Pay special attention to how your body feels within each stage of the pose and if the body feels tight or strained, release slightly. Always work with the body and not against it.

Mountainposture
Tadasana

As in the above image, stand straight, facing directly forward. Mountain posture is all about posture and have the body weight evenly distributed. Place the feet together, ensuring that your toes and heels are inline. The inside of your big toes and the centre of the inner ankles should touch lightly. Lift the soles of the feet from your mat, stretch them and then place them back down in the same position. Keep the toes down, stretching forwards. The weight must be distributed evenly on both the inner and outer edges of your feet as well as through the soles and heels. Keep the arches lifted. Extend up through the legs in a vertical manner as if stretching from the ankles through the Achilles tendons and up. Make sure that your legs remain facing forward and lock the knees, drawing the kneecaps softly up into the joints as if pulling from the outside in. Pull the thigh muscles up as if towards the top of the thighs.

Lift the hips and move the coccyx and sacrum forward, lengthening the spine and the trunk. The lower abdomen and abdominal organs should be up and back. Do not tense. Draw the buttock muscles upwards. Create space by lifting up the torso between the pelvis and the rib cage.

Move up through the body in this way, lifting the collarbones and opening up the chest by widening the front rips away from the sternum. Raise the upper chest and collarbones, drawing the skin of the shoulders towards the shoulder blades. The shoulder blades press down into the back.

Keep the shoulders relaxed and down and lengthen the neck. The upper arms should be turned outwards. Relax the arms and let them hang without tension. Often the neck and shoulders carry a great deal of tension, continue to extend the neck from below the shoulder blades without tensing the throat or the neck. Lift the back of the skull away from the neck, lightening the head. Your head should be straight and the chin level. Relax the face and look ahead. Stay in this pose for approximately 30 to 40 seconds, breathing evenly. Tadasana forms the starting pose for many postures and helps to prepare the mind and body for the posture to come.

Treepose
Vrksana

Stand in mountain pose (as previously) and prepare to move into Tree pose. Lift the right leg off the floor just slightly, standing firmly on the left leg. Place the left hand on the hip and bend the right leg now out to the side, taking the foot and pressing the sole into the very top of the inner left thigh. Try not to push the thigh out of alignment.

To keep the foot pressed against the left inner thigh, Harden the muscle. As you straighten the left knee, push the right knee outwards, so it is in line with the right hip. Lift the hip stretching up from the waist and through the chest. With balance solid, extend the arms to the sides turning the palms upwards, stretching both arms up over the head. Keep the elbows straight and feel the stretch through the sides of the body. The head must be straight and facing forward. Breath steadily and evenly. Hold this position for 20 to 30 seconds. Exhale and bring the arms down and then the right leg. Shake out both legs.

Repeat the process on the opposite leg

This posture aids balance and although it can be difficult initially, you can instruct your students to stand near a wall for support as this aids confidence. If they cannot join their palms together above the head with elbows straight, they should just keep the arms parallel. Balance can be improved by focusing on the placement of the foot and fixing the gaze.

Tip:
Make sure the shoulders are not hunched in the full extension of the arms
Triangle

UtthitaTrikonasana

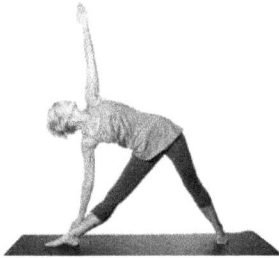

Therapeutic for:

Stretches the thighs, knees, and ankles
Stretches the hips, groins, hamstrings, and calves; shoulders, chest, and spine
Stimulates the abdominal organs
Helps relieve stress and improves digestion.
Helps relieve the symptoms of menopause
Relieves backache
Useful for the second stage of pregnancy
Eases neck pain, infertility, sciatica, osteoporosis
Alleviates anxiety.

Starting in Mountain pose, inhale, move the legs to hip width apart. Stretch the

arms out to the sides at shoulder level. The palms of the hands should be facing downwards. The feet should be in line but pointing forward. Visualise the extension of the soles and lift the arches. Now straighten the knees, stretching the shins and the knees upwards to the thighs. Raise the hips, work to extend the trunk up and open up the chest. The head should be kept straight. Elongate the arms right through to the thumbs and lock the elbows. Open the palms and focus your attention on stretching the fingers but keeping them together.
 From this position, turn the left foot inwards a little and turn the right leg 90° outwards so that the centre of the thigh, knee and the big toe point directly to the right. Adjust the feet so that the right heel is in line with the left arch. Press down the outer edge of the left foot and through the right inner heel and big toe. Lock the knees but do not strain.

Keep thigh muscles drawn upwards and arms extended. Be careful not to hold the breath. Inhale, then exhale and bend sideways as in the image. Bringing one arm down towards the knee (do not put pressure on the joint) and one arm upwards, pointing up to the ceiling, stretching through the fingers, moving the hips to the left, revolve the trunk and turn to look up to the hand. If any student has neck problems, keep the head facing forward. Hold this pose for 20 to 30 seconds and ensure breathing is normal throughout. Inhale, come up and return to the centre pose, then repeat on the other side.

Contraindications:

Diarrhea
Headaches

High blood pressure and low blood pressure   Neck   problems
Heart conditions

Warrior   pose   **Virabhadrasana   1**
Therapeutic for:

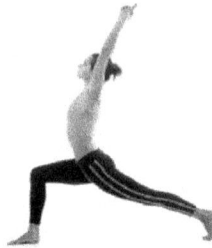

Stretches the chest and lungs, shoulders and neck, abdomen and groin area Strengthens the shoulders and arms. Strengthens the muscles of the back Strengthens and stretches the thighs, calves, and ankles

Stand in Mountain pose. Inhale and move the legs to approximately 4 feet apart with your arms stretched sideways. Turn the arms in their sockets so that the palms face upwards to the ceiling. Keep the arms straight, taking them over the head so they are parallel. At the same time as the arms extend upwards, stretch the sides of the chest and the armpits. Join the palms with the fingers stretching up, lock the elbows at this point. Turn the left foot 45 to 60° and the right foot 90° outwards, now turn the trunk to the right to face in the same direction as the right leg.

Turn the back of the leg and the hip together with the foot otherwise you may place a strain on the knees. Ensure that the feet are lined up. Both sides of the body should be parallel and then take the right hip just slightly backwards. Concentrate on the pubis, naval and sternum being centred and ensure your facing directly ahead which is to the right over the front foot. Take the waist back and then extend up with the trunk and arms in a vertical manner. Exhale, keeping the left leg firm, bending the right knee so that is at a right angle to the floor. The knees should still be facing directly forward. Keep the turn of the trunk and the lift of the hips as you move into this position. Then extend to the trunk upwards lifting the chest and throw the head back looking directly up.

Ensure that there is no strain on the throat or construction on the back of the neck. Stay in this position for 20 to 30 seconds and breath evenly throughout. Inhale and then straighten the knee and come back up to the centre. If required, the arms can be rested at this point. Then repeat on the other side.

Note: There is an extension of this posture i.e. Warrior 11 which can be studied once fitness and flexibility allows.
Contraindications:

High   blood   pressure
Heart   problems
Students with shoulder problems should keep their raised arms parallel (or slightly wider than parallel) to each other.
Students with neck problems should keep their head in a neutral position and not look up at the hands.

Reverse/Revolved   Triangle   **Parivrtta Trikonasana**

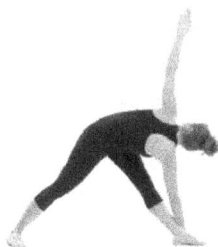

Therapeutic for:

Constipation
Digestionproblems
Sciatica
Lowerbackproblems
Asthma

Stand in Mountain pose and then move the legs to 4 feet apart on an inhalation. Arms stretched out sideways. The left leg and foot should be turned 45 to 60° inwards and the right leg 90° outwards. Ensure that the right heel is lined up with the left instep. Stretch the right leg and push back on the left leg. At the same time, bring the left hip and the left side of the trunk forward, taking the right side slightly back. Extend the trunk of the body upwards and keep the arms extended. The front of the body i.e. the pubis, naval and sternum now face directly forwards and the back of the body faces directly back. Press the left heel down and on an exhalation, swing the left side of the trunk down towards the right foot and turn the right side up extending the left arm from the shoulder so that the hand rests flat on the floor beside the outer edge of the right foot.

You can use the pressure of your fingers to be able to turn the trunk more. Keep the direction of the spine centred and let the trunk of the body follow the movement of the spine. Do not move the hips to one side. Extend the whole back right from the Coccyx up to the head, and work to revolve the hips, waist and chest. Strengthen the front of the body from the pubis right through the abdomen, chest and shoulders. Extend the right arm up turning your head as you do so and look upwards. Stay in this position for 20 to 30 seconds. Exhale and come out of the posture. Repeat on the other side once you have returned to the centre.

Contraindications:
This posture should be avoided if students suffer from:

Low   blood   pressure   Migraine
Diarrhoea
Headache
Insomnia

Standing   Forward   Bend   **Uttanasana**

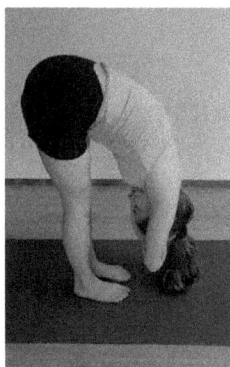

Therapeutic for:

Calming   the   brain.
Helps relieve stress and mild depression

Stimulates the liver and kidneys
Stretches hamstrings, calves, and hips
Strengthens the thighs and knees
Improves digestion
Helps alleviate symptoms of menopause
Reduces fatigue and anxiety
Improves sleep
Relieves headaches
Therapeutic for asthma, high blood pressure, infertility, osteoporosis, and sinusitis

This posture is wonderful to aid relaxation so that the body elongates in a passive way.

Stand in Mountain pose and then move the feet until they are about 1 foot apart. Clasp the elbows, inhale and stretched the arms over the head, take the elbows back. Now exhale, and take the trunk and the arms down towards the floor, extending from the hips so to avoid straining the lower back. Ensure the legs are stretched up and vertical. By pulling on the elbows, this extends the whole body down relaxing the head and neck. Let go of any tension.

In this position, ensure that the tops of the shin bones are stretched up and back. Stretch the knees up and imagine the bottom of the kneecaps tucking into the knee joints. Pull up the thigh muscles and press them back to grip the bones. Do not jerk the knees. All of the actions in and out of this posture should be smooth

 Contraindications: If a student has any back problems, advise them to bend their knees a little to take the pressure off the spine.

Dancers   Pose/   Lord   of   the   Dance

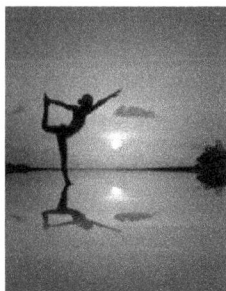

Therapeutic for:

Stretches   the   shoulders   and   chest
Stretches the thighs, groins, and abdomen

Strengthens legs and ankles Improves overall balance Adds a sense of grace

Stand in Tadasana (Mountain pose). Ensure that the body is facing straight ahead. Now, bend the right knee, lifting the foot behind towards the buttocks. Take hold of the ankle with the right hand. Steady the pose until ready to extend within the posture. On an inhalation, stretch the left arm up, keep the elbow straight and the arm close to the ear. The eyes should remain focussed on a point ahead to aid balance. Keep the right hand firmly on the ankle and now extend forward, stretching the right foot now away from the buttock. Raise the foot so that the right thigh is parallel to the ground. Hold the extended posture for as long as is comfortable, then shift the weight forward so that the chest and arm are parallel to the floor.

Note: The left arm should remain straight and close to the ear. The right arm is pulling against the right leg. Breathe normally throughout. Do watch that the standing leg does not bend and that the eyes are focussed on a stationery point ahead as this aids balance.

Balance improves quite quickly with regular practice and there are further extensions within this pose as flexibility improves.

Self-Assessment Test

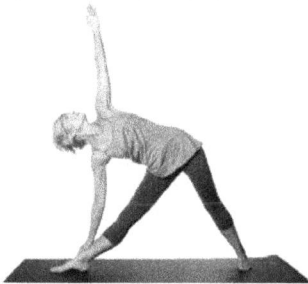

Task:
What is the Sanskrit word for Mountain Pose?
Task:
What are the contraindications for the Reversed Triangle Pose? Please note that these self-assessment

tasks are to ensure your understanding of the information within each module. As such, do not submit them for review with KEW Training Academy.

CHAPTER 19: PRACTICING YOGA AT HOME

Yoga offers innumerable benefits and certainly, the list of benefits increases manifold if it is practiced at homer, rather at health club, gum or studio. Yoga practices helps to make the person physically, mentally and spiritually fit, by promoting wellness, goodwill and harmony. It synchronizes our mind, body and soul and thus, fosters self-awareness and self-esteem. However, there are certain key points to determine, before commencing a yoga session at home. Firstly, identify and recognize the goal of practicing yoga at home. There are various different styles of yoga and mostly, people adopt yoga for a variety of reasons. This physical exercise offers stress management, healing and prevents ailments of our system. It even works on wellness components such as flexibility, strength, depression anxiety and stamina. The practice should be designed with keeping a close watch on the needs and requirements. Proper yoga technique, with a holistic goal, coupled with a strong motive, delivers excellent results. This would save you from the expensive membership plans of the gyms, studios and clubs and would render desirable results, as per your convenience. Secondly, yoga practice requires tranquil atmosphere. There should be enough space for moving, bending, backward, forward, and to the left and right. Your area should be spacious and well-ventilated. The room should be scented and with source of fresh air. If possible, try to experiment with Yoga in your own in-house Garden to immerse in the goodness of the environment. Thirdly, beginners need to purchase some yoga equipment, such as yoga mat and comfortable clothing from any local store.

Thirdly, purchasing some yoga DVD's is a good step for beginners, especially in the absence of proper and experienced guided practitioner .The choice of CD would depend again on your goal, needs and idea of Yoga. Videos may come in all ranges and would endorse various styles such as full body workout, fat burning, heat building and fast-paced postures. The videos may also be gentle, meditative, therapeutic and relaxing. Certain DVD is designed for various age groups and for various purposes. You can incorporate music with your yoga session. Hence, pick the DVD that best suits and fits your need. Fourthly, commence the Yoga routine by incorporating breathing exercise, warm-ups and meditation to relax and calm your mind. This technique is beneficial to help focus our attention. Adopt certain standing poses, twists, forward bends, twists, reclining poses and most crucial certain relaxation poses. Sixthly, make sure that you carry your yoga regime undisturbed and un-interrupted. Allot a time which is free from the buzzing of your phone and chaos of the daily routines. Design a specific timetable to surrender at least an hour to your yoga practice. You ought to spare at least devoting 5 to 7 days a week for yoga. Your frequency of practice would significantly affect, the results, you desire. As yoga is natural and side-effect free therapy, its regular practice would mean no harm and would only trigger mental, physical and psychological health.

CHAPTER 20: BASIC POSES

There are various reasons why adding yoga to your daily routine is healthy and beneficial. It improves flexibility; helps tone the muscles, enhance your balance and reduce your stress. Now that you are ready to give it a try, below are beginner poses also known as asanas for you to master.

SUKHASANA (Easy Cross Leg)

On a yoga mat, sit cross legged with your palms up, hand on your knees. Keep the spine straight while pushing the bones down on the floor or in yoga-speak, "sit bones". Keep your eyes closed and inhale. According to yoga experts, this is an ideal pose for beginners to do an assessment. Sitting on the floor allows you to feel and see the legs' external rotation. It is also good to relive stress and boosts the flexibility of your back.

MARJARYASANA/BITALASANA   (Cat-Cow Pose)

Get on the mat with your hands below your shoulders and knees below your hips. Equally distribute your weight on both hands and spread the fingers wide. Inhale and arch your back as you begin to lower your chin down to your chest. Exhale and lower your back to a scoop shape while you lift your head then tilt it back. This is good to address back pain and loosen the spine.

VRKASASANA (Tree Pose)

Begin by standing straight. Bring both the hands in a prayer position and life it over the head. Bend your left knee to the left side, press the left foot to your inner thigh while keeping you balance on your right leg. Hold this pose for 30 seconds then switch legs. It helps the body to stretch longer and also improves flexibility and balance. Apparently, the challenge here is to keep your balance in one leg. Poor balance is usually the result of a distracted mind. Moreover, this pose helps strengthen the claves, spine, ankles and thighs. It also helps reduce flat feet and stretches the shoulders and inner thighs.

BADDHA KONASANA (Bound Angle/Cobbler Pose) - is a usual sitting position of Indian cobblers. It improves general circulation by stimulating the heart. It also alleviates stress, anxiety, mild depression and fatigue. Sit straight while your legs are out in front. Bend your knees while pulling your heels toward the pelvis as you exhale. Drop your knees to the side and press your feet's soles. Do not force your knees. Stay in this pose for about 5 minutes then inhale. Lift your legs slowly away from the floor and go back to the original pose.

ADHO MUKHA SVANASANA (Downward Facing Dog Pose☐

Form your body to an inverted V-shape. Begin by placing the hands in front of you, palms down in your mat. It should be slightly in front of the shoulders. Put your knees on the ground under the hips. Lift your knees as you exhale and lift your hips and buttocks toward the ceiling. As you push your thighs back, stretch the heels toward the floor. Keep the head down between and inline the upper arms. You should be able to create a long spine. Likewise, this pose is a resting pose and the usual pose introduced to beginners. This also alleviates menopausal symptoms as well as menstrual discomfort.

BALASANA (Child's Pose)

Among the yoga poses, experts agreed that this is the most healing. The fetal position will make you feel relax. From the downward-facing dog pose, bend your knees while bringing your chest towards the floor. Lower the head and shoulders to the floor as well. Place both arms on your sides and palms up. Breathe in as you relax. This is an ideal post to stretch the back and release tensions.

TADASANA (Mountain Pose)

This pose is very simple as all you have to do is stand still with your hands broad at your side and your chest open. Feel the sensations in your back and legs and on your feet on the floor. It helps correct your posture, strengthen the thighs and feet and tone the muscles around the abdomen. Likewise, the mountain pose helps clear the mind, improves stability and balance.

There are other asanas that you can practice once you mastered these basic steps. Keep in mind that doing these poses should be comfortable for you or else, don't do it. Stop if it's painful and respect your body's limitations. The practice of yoga should be a pleasurable experience, not an excruciating one.

Chapter 21: Tips For Weight Loss, Overall Health, Happiness And Relieving Stress

In yogic philosophy, your eating habits do not only affect your physical well-being. Your mental capacities, emotional health and other vital energies are all influenced by the food you consume on a daily basis.

On Weight Loss

When did I last eat? – If your last meal is two to three hours ago, you probably aren't hungry and need not eat again. Remember, it takes the body at least 20 minutes to register a meal. If you have just eaten, allow yourself to have enough time to feel full.

Have I had enough to drink? – There are times when what feels like hunger is really just thirst. Eight glasses of water is recommended, and if you feel hungry for less than three hours after a meal, try drinking a glass of water.

Am I tired? – If you are over fatigue, you may be just looking for a quick pick-me-up. Try having a power nap rather than snacking on those bag of chips and bars of chocolates. You will be surprised at how refreshing the feeling is after a brief rest.

Am I under stress? – eating can be a form of comfort and release. If you think you have been stressing yourself out for the past days, try doing some light exercises. You may walk around your neighborhood or climb up the stairs. Make an effort to identify what triggers you to eat and your source of distress.

Am I too hard on myself? – pressuring yourself to lose weight at the soonest possible time is not going to be helpful at all. The more you burden yourself, the less likely you will lose those pounds. Learn to just control your portions and maintain a well-balanced diet.

How many hours of sleep do I have each night? – Sleeping is the body's way to rejuvenate and recharge in preparation for the next day's activities. Lack of sleep makes you gain weight for the simple reason that you tend to overeat especially the sugary and high-calorie comfort food.

On Health

Get moving – many are overweight not because they eat too much but because they exercise a little. Vigorous aerobic exercise – the kind that makes your heart beat faster and breathe deeper – is just what is needed. Keep in mind, the more energetically you move, the more calories you will burn.

The importance of strength training – you can build lean tissue by doing strength training. The more muscles you have, the more calories you burn. This comes from both a revved up metabolism and increased physical activity. Strengthening exercise likewise protects your muscles and bones so you won't lose lean tissue along with fat.

On the release of happy hormones – physical activity such as yoga helps trigger the release of mood-affecting chemicals in the body. These hormones, also known as endorphins, are responsible for the anti-depression and calming effect of exercise.

Maintain good posture –Proper posture avoids muscle strain and injury when you perform yoga poses – but that is just one of its benefits. The fastest way to look pounds lighter is when you stand tall. As your back and abdominals gets stronger, good posture becomes easier and second nature. And so whether you are sitting down or standing up, your body should always be relaxed but straight.

Believe in the power of slow starts and gradual but steady improvement – because there are good reasons to wait and not rush things. If you have been living a sedentary lifestyle, you probably have weak muscles. Weeks of yoga will improve all these. So do not feel overwhelmed at the first session. If you begin gradually and progress steadily, you can effortlessly ease yourself to a healthier lifestyle.

Try walking – this will help you stay fit and healthy, and it is much easier to include in your busy schedule. Try to sneak extra activity into your life by parking far away from where you are going, riding your bike for errands, and finding reasons to make multiple trips to the stairs.

Wake up your metabolism – even the simplest morning meal – say a bowl of cereal, skim milk and strawberries – lengthens attention span and elevates the mood until your next meal for the day. Studies say that breakfast eaters are slimmer ones because breakfast is the key component of weight control.

A workout buddy – have a standing appointment with a workout partner. If it is an always-there, can't-miss appointment, you will definitely do it. Having a workout buddy helps you become more motivated to exercise and change into a healthy lifestyle.

On Happiness and Stress Management

Focus – your thoughts may have the tendency to wander and jump around, but know that it is okay to not force your mind to be still. Pressuring your brain to do so will only stress you and set additional brain waves in motion. In order to manage your stress, just allow things to wander on your mind. And then gently command it to be calm and composed.

Cut out on alcohol – alcohol contains fermented ingredients and introducing toxins into the body will only result to a work up and stressed mind. Try to eliminate alcohol consumption from your diet in order to improve clarity and overall physical well-being.

Avoid too much caffeine – this is considered to be a powerful stimulant and causes the mind to be overactive thereby giving the body artificial energy. This also interrupts your normal sleeping pattern, spoiling your ability to slow down and rest.

The power of meditation – meditation is beneficial for people who are living stressful lives and continuing to find happiness in what they do. In meditation, the overactive and restless mind is calmed down and turned inward. This helps increase physical stamina, calmness and spiritual strength. Regular meditation produces a happier individual with a clearer mind and a deep sense of inner peace.

A more developed and relaxed patterns of behavior – yoga improves your concentration, manages stress and tension, and helps one achieve a more relaxed state. Try spending at least 30 minutes of yoga session each day. Regularity is key. Each session must begin with at least 5 minutes of relaxation, and must end with another 5 minutes rest.

Quell stress – uncontrolled stress can increase levels of the hormone cortisol, which is the one responsible in sending fat to the abdominal area. Exercise will help burn off stress hormones and may even

171

make you resistant to the effects of stress over time.

Sit down, close your eyes, and do some reflection – if you find stress overwhelming then take a moment to reflect and be grateful for what you have. Sit in silence and just be still. As you do so, make sure to clear your mind. If people would just allocate a few moments each day to reflect and be still, we will surely make for a happier, calmer and at peace society.

There is one particular exercise that you do in yoga that is particularly good for producing optimism, energy, zest for life and a real feeling of wellbeing. Practice it at home first but when you get accustomed to doing it, you can use this anyplace you want to and I would suggest that you practice it early in the morning in a place that you consider to be inspirational. This could be a beach area or you may want to hit the hills. Wherever you choose, be sure that you get an image of the skies and can see the sun coming up because this is your greeting to the sun or Sun Salutation. It is one of the mainstay yoga exercise routines that people use when they start their yoga practice for the day and it's a strong favorite with people who enjoy yoga.

Not only that, but it works on all the areas of your body to help get your chakras into alignment and help the flow of energy

173

through your body. Thus, practiced in the morning, this can add energy to your day.

The Sun Salutation

For the simple version of this which is suitable for beginners, stand on your mat and feel your body stretch, making sure that your legs are extended as your stand on flat feet and that your back is entirely straight. Bring your arms up above your head and reach toward the sky. Point your fingers toward the sky and feel the stretch of the body stretching onto your toes and then as you exhale bring your arms down by your sides and out in front of you to touch the area of the mat in front of your feet. Fold your head under so that it's tucked in, with your hands as nearly placed to your feet as you can get them. In the beginning stages of yoga before you have the strength and the bendability that you will gain with practice, you can bend your knees a little to achieve this position.

Straighten your arms and lift your body so that your back is flat and your head is lifted. As you exhale, move your legs back on the mat one big step with each leg until you are able to drop onto your knees and have bent elbows. Your hands should be flat on the mat at shoulder width and then you lean down into the mat so that your body is flat on the mat. Inhale and stretch your body, lifting the front part of your torso from the mat. Remember to tuck your feet so that you are resting on the balls of your feet and bring your body back up to the Downward Facing Dog position or inverted V that we practiced in the asana chapter.

On your next inhale, bring your legs back to the front of the mat so that you are standing folded in two with your head down like you were earlier in the exercise. Exhale and then inhale bringing yourself back to the standing position and sweep your arms up into the air and stretch, feeling the sky with the tips of your fingers.

Bring the arms down by your side and relax.

You can do this several times, but you need to get used to each of the movements before you race on through it. Remember that yoga is not about fast movements. It's about accuracy and about keeping your back straight and your tail area tucked in. It's about stretching to the limits without pain. If you need to bend, do so. Never force yourself.

The sun salutation that is performed in classes under supervision may be a little different to this because you have that supervision. However, when performing this on your own as a beginner, stick to the routine that is explained above as this gives you all the scope that you need. There are a few YouTube videos if you type in the words "Sun Salutation" and look for one that is for the beginner level.

The benefit of the sun salutation

This is a great exercise to start the day and to stretch you from sleeping, so that your body is alert and ready for anything. I also enjoy this at the end of the day because it's so helpful to sleeping. Your body doesn't feel strained and you actually feel like it's sufficiently relaxed if you take all the thoughts of the day out of the picture. Imagine living on a beach because this would be the perfect environment to do this last thing at night as that wonderful sun sinks against the horizon.

Most of us spend the day looking down at our phone or computer, sitting behind a desk, and slouching behind the wheel of a car. Because of this sedentary lifestyle we live, we tend to hold a lot of tension and pain in the neck. Since the neck is connected to everything else, tension in the neck can exacerbate arthritis pain in the shoulders and back. It can also cause debilitating headaches.

Those with arthritis pain in the neck know that this is one of the most painful places to have arthritis. When arthritis flares up in the neck, it gets in the way of living your life. Suddenly, you can't drive a car or even read a book without pain. These poses and exercises are gentle enough to bring a stretch to your neck when you are in pain, while helping to release tension and increase mobility.

Downward Facing Dog

Sanskrit name: Adho Mukha Svanasana

Downward Facing Dog is one of the most classic poses in the yoga canon. No yoga practice is complete without Down Dog. This pose delivers a full body stretch from your ankles to your neck. Dangling your neck between your hands allows the weight of your head to gently stretch and open up your neck.

If you have arthritis in your wrists or shoulders this pose may not be ideal. However, if you can work your way up to it, Down Dog can help to build muscles in the shoulders.

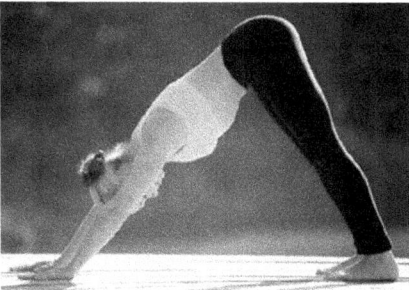

Instructions

Begin on your hands and knees in Tabletop Pose.

From there, tuck your toes and lift your hips into the air until your legs are as straight as you can comfortably get them. Those with very flexible ankles will be able to reach their feet to the floor, but most people will be on the balls of their feet.

Lengthen your tailbone towards the ceiling, spread your fingers wide, and move your shoulders down your back to create space for the neck to relax. Broaden your chest to create a stretch in the chest and upper back.

Breathe in this pose for as long as is comfortable.

Props

If your arms keep splaying outwards, this can put undue pressure on the shoulders. Loop a strap around your arms and pull it tight to keep your arms in alignment. You can press slightly against the strap to open the chest.

Modifications

If your wrist pain is too much to do this pose, try Dolphin Pose instead for a similar stretch.

To deepen the pose, alternate between bending your knees and drawing your right and left heel closer to the ground. This will deliver a deeper stretch to the calves.

Wide Legged Standing Forward Bend

Sanskrit name: Prasarita Padottanasana

Prasarita, as it is usually called, delivers the same benefits of a forward fold, but the wide-legged stance allows for a deeper stretch in the inner thigh. It also brings to the table the same calming benefits of inversion poses, but with none of the added tension to the neck, making this a great choice for those with neck pain.

On the topic of neck pain, this is a pose that allows the head to dangle freely,

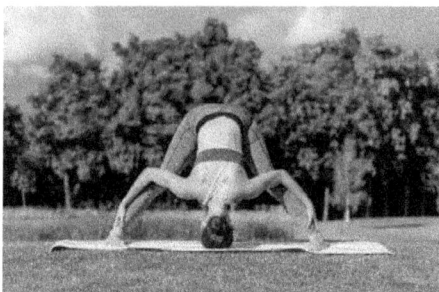

gently elongating and stretching the neck.

Instructions

Begin in Mountain Pose, then step one leg back about 3–4 feet.

Turn both feet so they are facing the same direction.

Fold forward until the crown of your head touches the earth, or as far as is comfortable.

You can keep your hands on your hips, reach them to the floor, or add in an arm posture for additional benefits.

Breathe in the pose as long as is comfortable.

Props

Many people are not able to reach their hands to the floor. In this case, you may place your hands on a block instead until you eventually work your way down to the floor.

Modifications

To deepen the shoulder stretch, add in a Hand Clasp or Reverse Prayer Hands.

Modified Fish Pose

Sanskrit name: Matsyasana

Fish Pose is an intense back bend that really opens up the throat and neck. It might be a little too intense for beginners and those suffering from neck pain, so this modified version is a better option. This pose is amazingly relaxing, so add it towards the end of your practice or before bed. The front body stretch also provides fantastic relief for backaches, tight hips, digestive issues, and respiratory issues. If you also are struggling with autoimmune disease, that powerful combination makes this an ideal pose for you.

If you have a migraine, however, this pose is best avoided.

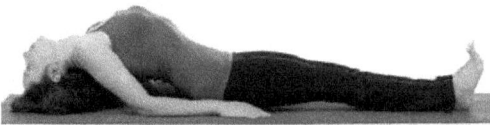

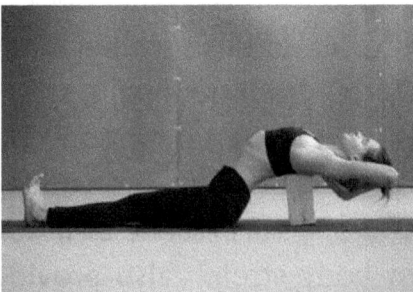

Instructions

Begin by lying on your back on your yoga mat with two blocks (or one block and a pillow) within arms' reach.

Inhale and lift your chest slightly. Insert a block on its side between your shoulder blades. Bend backwards over the block.

If this is too much for your neck, insert another block or a pillow beneath your head to take some of the pressure off.

Breathe deeply in this pose, allowing each breath to open the chest. Hold the posture for as long as needed.

Cat and Cow Poses

Sanskrit name: Marjaryasana/Bitilasana

Cat/Cow Pose is actually two separate postures that are usually done in rounds, one after the other. Combined, they're a yoga classic; rarely will you leave a yoga class without doing Cat/Cow.

Cat Pose provides a stretch to the upper back, massages your internal organs, and allows the neck to hang loose and relax. Cow Pose stretches the front of the neck and broadens the chest, while likewise massaging your organs and spine.

This combination of poses gently warms up the neck and the spine, so it's best added in at the beginning of your yoga practice to release tension and prepare for more intense poses. The stretch to the front body and gentle massage of the stomach organs makes these poses a powerful tonic for digestive issues, so add the pair into your routine if you're struggling with autoimmune symptoms.

Cow Pose

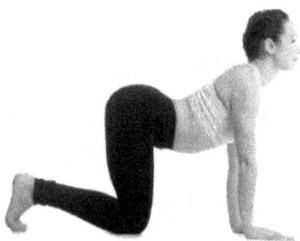

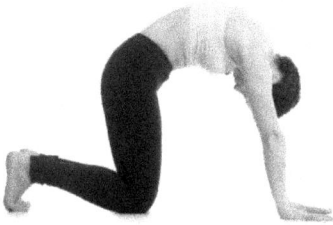

Cat Pose

Instructions

Begin in Tabletop Pose.

On the inhale, arch your back downward, lift your chest and head, and lift your tailbone slightly to the sky. This is Cow Pose.

On the exhale, round your spine high, lowering your head and allowing it to dangle. Allow your neck to relax into Cat Pose.

Repeat this cycle as many times as needed.

Props

If you are unable to rest on your knees, try adding a blanket or gel pads beneath them.

Modifications

If your knees are still too sore, you can practice this pose standing up against a wall. Put your hands against the wall and mimic the movement of the postures.

Rag Doll

Sanskrit name: Baddha Hasta Uttanasana

Rag Doll Pose, also known as Dangling Pose, is one of those super relaxing postures that's the perfect tonic for stress. This pose allows you to dangle your head to the ground, elongating your neck, and saying goodbye to tension in the neck and shoulders. It also provides a delicious stretch to your upper back and legs.

Because this pose is so simple, you can do it any time you need a break. This is the perfect pose to do behind your desk when your neck and back are hurting from looking down at your computer screen all

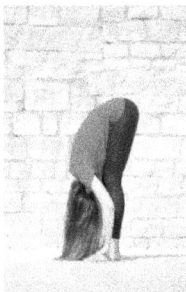

day.

Instructions

Begin in Mountain Pose, with your feet hip distance apart.

Drape your entire body forward. Bend your knees slightly to reduce pressure on the knees. If your legs are very stiff, bend your knees as much as needed.

You may rest your hands on the ground, or grasp opposite elbows.

Allow your head to hang and your neck to become elongated.

Breathe in this pose for as long as is needed.

Modifications

To enhance the shoulder stretch, bend your knees until your chest is resting against your upper legs, then add a Hand Clasp behind your back.

Standing Split

Sanskrit name: Urdhva Prasarita Eka Padasana

Standing Split is a kind of forward bend, so it allows your neck to release. This pose also stretches the entire leg and opens up the hips, while calming the mind. It's an inversion, making this a fantastic way to release tension from the entire body at the end of the day.

Standing Split also forces you to balance ever so slightly. Balancing poses provide a gentle workout to your core. Strengthening your core is key to preventing the injuries and lower back

pain that come with arthritis and

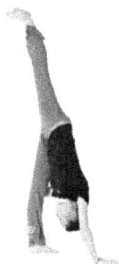

osteoporosis.

Instructions

Begin in Mountain Pose.

Bring your hands down to the mat and place your palms flat on the earth on either side of your right foot.

Spread your fingers for stability.

Lift your left leg towards the sky. You may only be able to get your leg up a few inches, but over time you'll be able to reach your leg higher.

Activate your leg and turn your toes down to the ground.

Ensure that your standing leg is not collapsing inwards.

Release your neck and allow gravity to gently pull on your head.

Breathe in this pose for as long as is comfortable, then repeat it on the other side.

Props

Support the lifted leg on a chair if this pose is too intense.

If your hands cannot reach the ground, place both hands on a block.

Modifications

Focus your gaze on a still point on the ground to help balance.

To deepen the pose and challenge your balance, grasp your hands around your standing ankle.

Camel Pose

Sanskrit name: Ustrasana

Camel Pose can be pretty intense for beginners, so it's best to work your way up to this pose. Even if you've been doing yoga for a long time, Camel Pose is something you'll want to add in towards the end of your practice, once your neck and back have had the chance to warm up.

Camel Pose provides a deep stretch to the neck, throat, chest, shoulders, and stomach, so this pose can practically be a panacea for all of your body aches. The gentle stretch to the stomach also helps to alleviate the digestive discomfort caused by autoimmune disorders or heavy painkillers.

If you have a neck injury, knee pain, or a migraine, this pose should be skipped.

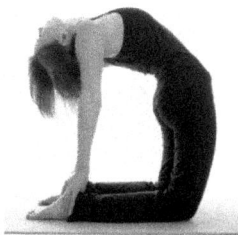

Instructions

Kneel on your mat with your knees hip distance apart.

Breathe in as you lengthen your entire body upwards, stretching the crown of your head towards the sky and elongating your neck.

Place your hands on your lower back, open your chest, lean your head backwards, and release your neck.

You can rest here or deepen the pose by reaching your hands further backwards to grab your heels.

Shut your eyes and breathe in a comfortable position for as long as needed, then release the pose.

Props

This pose might be tough on your knees. If you have sore knees, fold a blanket or your mat beneath them.

Dolphin Pose

Sanskrit name: Makarasana

Like in Downward Facing Dog Pose, in Dolphin Pose your neck is able to hang freely, allowing gravity to deliver a gentle stretch to the neck. Dolphin Pose does, however, grant a more intense stretch to other parts of the body than Downward Facing Dog does. In Dolphin Pose, your upper back will also feel a major release, allowing your neck even more relief. If you sit behind a computer all day, you definitely need to add Dolphin Pose in to your routine to release the tension in your neck that makes arthritis pain so much worse.

A word of caution, this pose might be a little too intense if you have arthritis in your shoulders. Instead, work your way up to this pose and follow the instructions

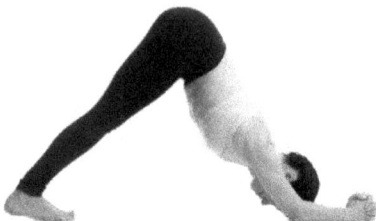

carefully to avoid injuring your shoulders.

Instructions

From Tabletop Pose, lower onto your forearms. Your hands should be flat against your mat, with your fingers engaged and reaching out for stability.

Engage your arms and lift your hips until your hips are in the air and you are resting on the balls of your feet, like in Downward Facing Dog.

Make sure your shoulders are aligned with your elbows, and your elbows are not moving out to the side, to prevent shoulder injury.

Engage your legs to take the pressure off of your shoulders.

Take 5–10 breaths in this pose and allow your neck to dangle freely.

Slowly come down to your knees when you are ready to exit the pose.

Upward Plank Pose

Sanskrit name: Purvottanasana

Not only does Upward Plank Pose help to release tension in the neck, it also opens up the entire front body, creating space where there used to just be tension. It's an excellent way to counterbalance sitting all day long. This pose does, however, provide more of a challenge than more restorative poses, so it's best to work your way up to this pose; do not begin with it right away.

If you're recovering from a back injury, this pose might not be the best for you. But if you want to create more flexibility in your back, Upward Plank Pose is a great way to prepare for more intense backbends.

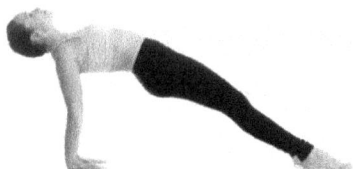

Instructions

Begin sitting on the ground with your legs in front of you.

Your hands should be slightly behind your buttocks, no more than shoulder width apart. Your fingers should be pointing towards your feet.

Slowly begin to lift your hips with the soles of your feet planted on the ground. Your feet should be about hip width apart.

Lift your chest up and allow your neck to slowly release backwards.

Take 3–5 breaths in this pose and release.

Modifications

If this pose is too difficult, you can practice Reverse Tabletop Pose instead. In Reverse Tabletop, you bend your knees at a 90-degree angle instead of fully extending your legs.

If this pose puts too much of a strain on your neck, practice with your head resting on a chair or against the wall.

If your wrists are too sore for this pose, just skip it and practice Cobra Pose or Sphinx Pose against a chair.

CHAPTER 24: THE DIFFERENCE BETWEEN YOGA AND MINDFULNESS

The reason why mindfulness is so important in your learning of yoga is that although it's a totally different discipline, it helps you to develop confidence and to be able to more accepting of what happens to you within your life. Used in conjunction with yoga it's extremely powerful. Yoga is the discipline of using different positions to free up the chakras, but mindfulness opens the mind so if you can do both in conjunction with each other, imagine the power that you are embracing. It really is powerful.

As the quotation above says, mindfulness means being mindful. It means noticing things around you but not actually having an opinion of the things that you see. That means that you can accept what is happening – whether this goes in your favor or not – and are able to look at life from a much wider viewpoint. It also means noticing things. You notice when the buds turn into leaves. You notice when a petal falls from a rose in the garden. You notice the taste and texture of whatever hits your tongue during a meal and you begin to hone in on your senses to see things that perhaps you never took the time to notice in the past. It's important because the only moment that you live in is this moment. There's no point in looking back with regret because when you do that, you waste this moment in negativity. In a similar manner, looking forward to something with dread and worry is pointless because it hasn't happened yet. Mindfulness embraces the moment, and there can be no better yoga pose to make you feel the benefit of mindfulness than the sun salutation.

If you are able to practice this in a very inspiring place, such as a beach or a natural beauty spot, it uplifts you and makes you feel that the world is a very precious place to be. In fact, you may even have seen a yoga class doing this on the beach and it's an extremely useful exercise to get all of your body feeling alive and ready to take on the world.

Sun Salutation for Beginners

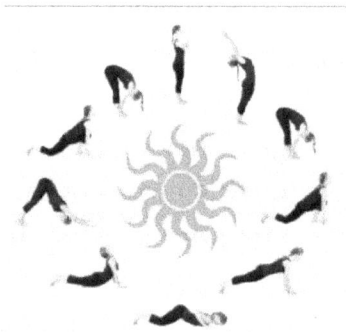

Stand with your feet at shoulder width and breathe easily. Don't force the breath at all, and move the arms out to the sides turning the hands so that they face upward. Exhale, and bring the hands into the prayer position. Inhale and then reach your hands as far as you can reach them up to the sky. Exhale and lean forward so that you are bending at the waist and so that your arms reach out to the sides before coming down in front of you in a swan movement. Keeping your hands on your ankles inhale and lean your head forward. Exhale and then move your left leg out behind you followed by your right leg so that you are supporting your body on the flat hands and the balls of your feet.

Breathe deeply so that the breath goes into your chest. Bend your elbows so that your body goes flat on the floor but keep your hands on the mat. Straighten your arms so that you are looking upward in an upward facing dog position. Then put your feet flat on the floor and pull your body up into an inverted V or downward facing dog position. While in this position breathe for a few moments as this helps the flow of energy through your body.

Inhale and move your foot forward between your hands, looking forward as you do so. Bring your other leg forward so you are bent and bring your arms out to the side. Then take a deep breath and bring your hands up to as high as you can get them above your head. Go back into the prayer position with your hands together in front of you. Relax.

This exercise is very useful for stretching the back and keeping your posture. Pay close attention to the breathing as you do this exercise. You won't get it right at first but it's a very strange feeling when you do because your body, your mind and your breathing all work in unison and it feels very right.

There are distinct differences between yoga and mindfulness but if you use mindfulness during your poses, what you find happens is that there is a better flow to your movements and you are more conscious of your breathing and able to find the right harmony of all of these facets that make your yoga a natural extension to the movements that you make in general. You will feel the energy because of your mindfulness and so the two disciplines go hand in hand to give you a fuller experience.

Conclusion

Yoga, if practiced regularly can help you live a harmonious and beautiful life. Use the yoga poses described in this book to become healthy, happy, and calm.

Thank you again for downloading this book!

I hope this book was able to help you to know all that you need to know about yoga as a beginner.

The next step is to start practicing what you have learnt and see a change in your life.

Thank you and good luck!